Common Symptoms
DESCRIBED FOR NURSES

BY JOHN GIBSON

MD, FRCPsych

SECOND EDITION

BLACKWELL SCIENTIFIC PUBLICATIONS
OXFORD LONDON EDINBURGH MELBOURNE

© **1976, 1978** Blackwell Scientific Publications
Osney Mead, Oxford
John Street, London WC1
9 Forrest Road, Edinburgh
P.O. Box 9, North Balwyn, Victoria, Australia

First published 1976
Second edition 1978

British Library Cataloguing in Publication Data

Gibson, John, b.1907
    Common symptoms described for nurses. — 2nd ed.
    1. Semiology   2. Nursing
    I. Title
    616.07'2'024613   RT65
    ISBN 0-632-00442-8

Distributed in the United States of America by
J.B. Lippincott Company, Philadelphia
and in Canada by
J.B. Lippincott Company of
Canada Ltd, Toronto

Printed in Great Britain by
Billing & Sons Limited,
Guilford, London and Worcester.

Contents

Introduction

This book is to help a nurse when she first meets a patient in an out-patient clinic or in a ward. He will come with a symptom or with several symptoms. By referring to the appropriate sections in the book the nurse may quickly inform herself of the likely cause of the patient's complaints and can then turn to her textbook of medicine or surgery to inform herself further.

Preface to Second Edition

For the second edition this book has been revised throughout. Two new sections have been added: one on Nasal Catarrh, the other on Pain and Lumps in the Breast.

1. Pyrexia

The temperature is regulated by a centre in the hypothalamus of the brain. The centre reacts to the blood passing through it. Taken in the mouth and rectum, the temperature recorded indicates the 'core temperature' of the body, i.e. that of thoracic and abdominal organs and of the brain. The mouth temperature is normally in the range 36·0°–37·5°C (97·0°–99·5°F); the rectal temperature is slightly higher. Temperature recorded in the axilla and groin is slightly lower. There is a normal daily variation, with the temperature being highest in the afternoon and lowest in the small hours; the pattern is not altered in a night worker. The temperature is higher in the premenstrual period in women than in the post-menstrual period.

Pyrexia is a rise of temperature above the normal range. It is most commonly due to the action on the temperature-regulating centre of pyrogens, chemical substances discharged in tiny amounts into the blood by the action of micro-organisms and from diseased tissues.

PUO means Pyrexia of Unknown Origin, and is a term commonly used until the cause of a pyrexia is discovered.

Daily variation. In most fevers the temperature is higher at night than in the morning. It can be higher in the morning than at night in some cases of:

> typhoid fever,
> tuberculosis,
> meningococcal infection.

Rigors. Rigors are shivering attacks with a feeling of cold which occur in some fevers when the superficial surface of the body is cold while the core temperature is rising sharply. The shivering is due to involuntary muscular contractions. Rigors can be a feature of:

> malaria,
> septicaemia,
> pyaemia,

1

the onset of a pneumococcal pneumonia,
E. coli infections of the urinary tract,
cholangitis.

Causes of pyrexia

Infections
Neoplasms
Hypersensitivity reactions
Disturbance of temperature-regulating mechanisms
Circulatory disturbances
Other causes

Infections

Pyrexia can be caused by bacterial, viral, protozoal, and metazoal infections.

Pyrexia can be:

(a) continuous: the temperature is raised continuously above the normal and does not vary more than 1°C in 24 hours,

(b) intermittent: the temperature falls to normal at least once in 24 hours,

(c) remittent: the temperature varies more than 1°C in 24 hours but does not fall to normal,

(d) periodic: bouts of fever are separated by afebrile periods of several days. This occurs in:

> malaria,
> relapsing fever,
> brucellosis,
> rat-bite fever,
> some cases of Hodgkin's disease (Pel-Ebstein fever),
> systemic lupus erythematosus.

Neoplasms

Pyrexia can occur in any rapidly advancing malignant disease, as a result of a discharge of pyrogens from damaged cells or from a secondary infection. It is commonly a feature of:

hypernephroma: a malignant tumour of the kidney most common in the first two years of childhood,

carcinoma of the liver: due to secondary deposits from a primary elsewhere, e.g. the stomach, the large intestine, the breast,

lymphosarcoma: a malignant tumour of lymph tissue.

Pyrexia can also occur in:

Hodgkin's disease (lymphadenoma): fever can be of the Pel-Ebstein type with afebrile periods between bouts,

acute leukaemia: fever is associated with enlarged lymph nodes, enlarged spleen, anaemia, purpura and haemorrhages from the gums and intestinal tract,

myelomatosis (multiple myeloma): a malignant proliferation of plasma cells; infections are common owing to an inability to form antibodies,

fibroid tumour of the uterus: pyrexia can occur with red degeneration of a fibroid.

Hypersensitivity reactions

Pyrexia can be due to a hypersensitivity to drugs or foreign proteins, and is likely to be associated with urticaria, itching, vomiting, pains in the limbs and albuminuria. The pyrexia and other features may be delayed for 24 hours to 14 days.

(a) *Drugs.* Drugs particularly liable to cause pyrexial attacks in sensitive people include:

> penicillin,
> cephalosporin,
> chloramphenicol,
> sulphonamides.

(b) *Foreign proteins.* Pyrexia due to foreign proteins can follow the injections of:

> sera,
> vaccines,
> blood.

Collagen diseases

Pyrexia can be a symptom of:

(a) *systemic lupus erythematosus* (SLE) in which a periodic fever is likely to be associated with a butterfly rash on the face, painful swollen joints, and loss of weight.

(b) *polyarteritis nodosa*, in which fever is likely to be associated with limb pains, abdominal pain and a raised pulse rate due to inflammatory changes in medium-sized and small arteries.

Disturbances of temperature-regulating mechanisms

The mechanisms by which temperature is controlled can be disturbed in various conditions with the result that a state of hyperpyrexia is produced. This can happen in:

(a) *heat stroke*: due to long continuous exposure to intense heat as in a desert or in a very hot engine-room.

(b) *lesions of the hypothalamus*: the temperature-regulating centre is disturbed or destroyed.

(c) *ichthyosis*: due to the disease of the skin there is inadequate heat-loss from the surface of the body.

Circulatory disturbances

(a) *Mycocardial infarcation* (due to coronary thrombosis): a mild fever commonly begins on the first or second day and a lasts for a few days.

(b) *Pulmonary infarction*: fever may or may not occur.

(c) *Thrombophlebitis*: fever usually occurs in this condition in which the veins of the leg become thrombosed, palpable and tender.

(d) *Subarachnoid haemorrhage*: a slight rise of temperature may occur about 24 hours after the onset and last for a week.

Other causes

(a) *Crohn's disease*: fever is common and due either to the disease itself or to secondary abscesses. Other features are likely to be abdominal pain, diarrhoea, and loss of weight.

(b) *Thyroid crisis*: a sudden flooding of the circulation with thyroid hormones causes pyrexia, confusion, diarrhoea and a rapid pulse; it can occur as a complication of thyrotoxicosis or after thyroidectomy in an inadequately prepared patient.

(c) *Dental sepsis*: prolonged fever, malaise and sometimes joint pains can be caused by dental sepsis and cured by appropriate dental treatment.

2. Loss of Weight

Loss of weight may in some conditions be associated with:
    vitamin deficiency,
    protein deficiency,
    dehydration.

Oedema can hide loss of essential tissues because the oedematous fluid weighs as much as or more than the tissue lost.

Causes of loss of weight

Deficient intake of food
Malabsorption syndromes
Infections
Neoplasms
Endocrine abnormalities
Parasites

Deficient intake of food

Deficient intake of food may be due to:

(a) starvation: the person cannot get enough to eat.

(b) voluntary reduction: the person has decided to slim.

(c) alcoholism: chronic alcoholism causes chronic gastritis and cirrhosis of the liver which reduces the appetite.

(d) drug addiction: appetite is lost.

(e) old age: deficient intake may be due to poverty, senility, inability to go shopping or to cook, or to ill-fitting dentures.

(f) depression: the person is too depressed to eat, thinks it is wicked to eat or be alive, is deluded that he cannot digest food or has no bowels, or attempts suicide by starvation.

Malabsorption syndromes

The patient may take an adequate diet, but because of disease of the small intestine he cannot absorb foodstuffs and consequently loses weight.

Common conditions which cause malabsorption are:

(a) *Idiopathic steatorrhoea* (non-tropical sprue: called coeliac disease in children). Due to hypersensitivity to gluten, the child when he starts to eat bread loses his appetite and has diarrhoea and a distended abdomen. The condition continues into adult life.

(b) *Crohn's disease* (regional ileitis). Loss of weight is associated with abdominal pain, diarrhoea, and masses in the abdomen due to a chronic inflammatory state of the small intestine and sometimes of the large intestine.

(c) *Surgical operations on the small intestine.* Malabsorption can be due to surgical removal of a length of small intestine so that what is left is too short for proper absorption to take place. Volvulus or infarction are the usual reasons for such a removal.

If an operation (such as partial gastrectomy with gastro-enterostomy) has left a blind-ended loop of bowel or when disease of the small intestine has caused strictures or fistulae between loops of intestine, the contents of the loop can become stagnant, the number of bacteria in it increases, and there is interference with the absorption of foodstuffs; this is called the stagnant loop syndrome.

(e) *Deficiency of pancreatic juice.* Pancreatic juice is essential for the digestion of foodstuffs. Lack of it causes malabsorption. A deficiency of pancreatic juice can be due to:

> pancreatitis,
> carcinoma of the pancreas,
> fibrocystic disease of the pancreas.

Pancreatitis and carcinoma of the pancreas occur in adult life. Fibrocystic disease occurs in early childhood.

(f) *Deficiency of bile salts.* Bile salts are essential for the digestion of fat. Lack of them cause malabsorption. A deficiency of bile salts can be due to:

hepatitis,
obstruction of the bile duct by gall-stones or by
carcinoma of the head of the pancreas.

Infections

Loss of weight can occur in any acute or chronic infection. It
is particularly likely to be a feature of:

tuberculosis,
bacterial endocarditis,
chronic sepsis,
malaria,
brucellosis.

Neoplasms

Loss of weight occurs in any malignant condition. It is likely
to be an early feature of

carcinoma of the oesophagus,
carcinoma of the stomach.

Endocrine diseases

Loss of weight is a feature of certain endocrine diseases.

(a) *Simmonds' disease.* Loss of weight follows loss of appetite
and is associated with fatigue, pallor, amenorrhoea and
degeneration of the genitalia. The condition is due to a
degeneration of the pituitary gland and a failure of pituitary
hormonal secretion.

(b) *Diabetes insipidus.* Loss of weight is due to loss of fluid
owing to enormous amounts of urine being excreted. In this
condition there is failure of ADH (anti-diuretic hormone)
secretion with the result that the renal tubules do not reabsorb
the fluid they should.

(c) *Hyperthyroidism.* Loss of weight is associated with
anxiety, tremor, a rapid pulse and an enlarged thyroid gland.
The condition is due to an excessive production of thyroid
hormones.

(d) *Diabetes mellitus.* Loss of weight occurs in severe, inadequately treated diabetes. Associated features are likely to be

an excessive secretion of urine, thirst, dehydration and ketosis.

(e) *Addison's disease.* Loss of weight is likely to be associated with fatigue, nausea, vomiting and pigmentation of the skin. The condition is due to a failure of secretion of hormones by the adrenal cortex.

Parasites

Loss of weight and anaemia can occur with infection by:

  ancylostoma (hookworm),
  giardia lamblia
  schistosomiasis (bilharzia).

3. Fatigue

The patient may complain of fatigue, tiredness or debility.

Causes of fatigue

Mental states
Anaemia
Infection
Endocrine abnormalities
Malabsorption syndromes
Hypertension
Chronic renal failure
Chronic lead poisoning

Mental States

(a) *Boredom* can masquerade as fatigue. The person who is bored with his job, is not intellectually stimulated by his work or other activities, or is left alone for long periods can complain of fatigue.

(b) *Simple schizophrenia.* In this form of schizophrenia the patient is usually a young man or woman who drifts, is devoid of drive, grows detached from reality, and may complain of fatigue or vague hypochondriacal complaints.

(c) *Hysteria.* Fatigue may be a hysterical conversion symptom in a person who shows other evidence of hysteria.

Anaemia

Anaemia of any type is likely to produce fatigue. The patient is likely to be pale and may complain of shortness of breath or precordial pain on exertion. The anaemia may be:

iron-deficiency anaemia,
pernicious anaemia,
haemolytic anaemia,

aplastic anaemia,
thalassaemia (due to blood loss)

or may occur in:

leukaemia,
Hodgkin's disease (lymphadenoma),
myelomatosis (multiple myeloma).

Infection

Any chronic, mild or unsuspected infection or inflammatory process can cause fatigue. Particular conditions of which fatigue may be an early feature are:

tuberculosis of any organ,
bacterial endocarditis,
urinary infection,
typhoid fever in the first week,
brucellosis,
sarcoidosis.

Depression and fatigue are common after influenza.

Endocrine abnormalities

Fatigue can be a symptom of:

hypothyroidism,
Addison's disease,
diabetes mellitus.

(a) *Hypothyroidism.* Fatigue due to hypothyroidism (myx-oedema) is likely to be associated with constipation, stiffness of muscles, intolerance of cold, oedema of face and legs, pallor with a malar flush, impaired mental functioning and a croaky voice. The patient is likely to be over the age of thirty.

(b) *Addison's disease.* Fatigue is likely to be associated with loss of weight, pigmentation of the skin, nausea and vomiting, vague abdominal discomfort and dehydration. The patient is likely to be an adult. The disease is due to a failure of production of hormones by the cortex of the adrenal glands.

(c) *Diabetes mellitus.* Fatigue can be an early symptom of diabetes mellitus, especially in the mild, mature-onset type of the disease which occurs in overweight middle-aged or old people.

Malabsorption syndromes

Fatigue is likely when a patient is unable to absorb the food he eats. Failure of absorption can be due to:

> idiopathic steatorrhoea,
> Crohn's disease,
> disease of the pancreas,
> disease of the liver or bile-ducts,
> surgical interference with the small intestine.

There is likely to be a failure of absorption of fat, iron, calcium, potassium, salt and vitamins. Fatigue is particularly likely to be due to a failure to absorb adequate amounts of potassium and salt.

Hypertension

Fatigue is a symptom of hypertension (raised blood pressure) and is likely to be associated with headache (the predominating symptom) and in severe cases with palpitations, breathlessness on exertion and giddiness.

Chronic renal failure

Fatigue is a symptom of chronic renal failure (uraemia). There is likely to be a known history of kidney disease. Fatigue is associated with nausea, vomiting, hiccough, a dry tongue, a yellowish pigmentation of the skin, depression and confusion.

Chronic lead poisoning

Fatigue, headache, indigestion, abdominal discomfort, diarrhoea or constipation, and a pallor with a slightly yellow tinge are early features of chronic lead poisoning, which can occur in some industrial processes.

4. Headache

Headache can be due to conditions within the skull, conditions outside the skull, general diseases of the body or psychological causes. The brain and bones of the skull are insensitive; the periosteum is sensitive. Headache can in some conditions be due to dilatation and to contraction of intercranial or extra-cranial blood vessels and to displacement of the venous sinuses in the dura matter.

Causes of headache

Muscle tension
Migraine
Periodic migrainous headache
Hypertension
Raised intracranial pressure
Reduced intracranial pressure
Stroke
Transient ischaemic attacks
Meningitis
Trauma
Cranial arteritis
Pyrexia
Alcohol and some drugs

Muscle tension headache (nervous headache, psychogenic headache)

This is a common type of headache and is produced by anxiety, depression, aggression and frustration. It occurs in the frontal, temporal, parietal and occipital regions and in the neck. It can be unilateral or bilateral. It may be a dull ache or a feeling of constriction or pressure. It is attributed to long-sustained contraction of the frontalis and occipital muscles in the scalp or of muscles in the face and neck. There may be

13

tender or painful spots in the scalp, and wearing a hat or brushing the hair can be painful. The headache is sometimes further increased by dilatation of the cranial arteries.

Migraine

Attacks of migraine start in childhood, in girls often at the start of menstruation. The headache of migraine is usually limited to one side of the head, but it is sometimes generalized or present in the front or back of the head only. It is preceded by visual symptoms—mistiness of vision, spots, coloured stars or fortification figures (like plans of old forts)—which last for up to three-quarters of an a hour. The headache begins as the visual symptoms fade and becomes intense. It usually lasts for several hours, after which the patient falls asleep. Sometimes it lasts for days. It is associated with giddiness, nausea and vomiting. During the attack the patient is pale; and the superficial temporal artery may be thickened and pulsating strongly. There may be a feeling of depersonalisation the day after an attack.

Several variations of the classical migraine occur:

(a) *basilar artery migraine*: this variety occurs usually in adolescent girls in whom the pain occurs only in the occipital region.

(b) *hemiplegic migraine*: severe unilateral headache is followed by hemiparesis or hemiplegia on the opposite side of the body. The paralysis clears up in up to 10 days.

(c) *opththalmic migraine*: headache is concentrated around one eye and is followed by paralysis of the oculomotor (third cranial) nerve and sometimes of all the motor nerves to the eye on the same side.

Periodic migrainous neuralgia

This neuralgia differs from migraine in that:

(a) it starts later in life, usually in middle age,

(b) an attack starts in the middle of the night,

(c) the pain is always unilateral; it begins in the eye and spreads to the forehead and temporal region and sometimes into the neck,

(d) the affected eye is red and weeps profusely,

(e) visual disturbances and vomiting are uncommon,

(f) the patient is restless in the attack and paces up and down.

Hypertension

(a) *Benign hypertension.* Attacks of headache can vary from mild to severe, and can be associated with palpitations, nervousness and giddiness. Some patients with benign hypertension do not get headache.

(b) *Malignant hypertension.* Headache is usually severe and lasts up to a day at a time. It may be generalized or localized to the top or front of the head. It is often accompanied by nausea and vomiting.

(c) *Hypertensive encephalopathy.* Due to a steep rise of an already high BP, the patient develops a sudden, splitting headache with vomiting and drowsiness and sometimes fits and unconsciousness. An attack lasts for hours or days before clearing up, and can recur.

Raised intracranial pressure

Headache occurs in most cases of raised intracranial pressure. A raised intracranial pressure can be due to:

> tumour of the brain,
> tumour of the auditory (eighth cranial) nerve, meninges or skull,
> abscess of brain,
> hydrocephalus in an adult.

At first the headache is not very severe. It is usually present on waking and worst in the morning. It starts by being paroxysmal and goes on to become continuous. It is usually generalized, but it can be localized to one side or to the front, top or back of the head; when it is unilateral, it is not necessarily on the same side as the lesion. It tends to throb with the pulse and is made worse by coughing, sneezing, stooping and straining. Vomiting without nausea is likely. Drowsiness, excessive sleep, memory defects and slow mental processes are commonly present.

Reduced intracranial pressure

Headache can be due to a reduction in intracranial pressure after a lumbar puncture if the patient is allowed to sit up or stand immediately afterwards. It is prevented and relieved by lying down.

Stroke

A very severe headache can occur as the first symptom of a cerebral haemorrhage, thrombosis or embolism, and occur before the onset of paralysis and coma.

With a berry aneurysm of the circle of Willis, leakage of blood may have caused earlier attacks of milder headache with stiffness of the neck.

Transient ischaemic attacks

These attacks come on suddenly, last for 24 hours and leave no residual signs. They are due to the passage of an embolus through the internal carotid or vertebral artery. In about 25 per cent of cases headache occurs during or after an attack. When the embolus is in the internal carotid artery or one of its branches, the headache is usually frontal or temporal and is accompanied by unilateral weakness of the face, arm or leg, sometimes with speech disturbance or impairment of vision. When the embolus is in the vertebral artery or one of its branches, headache is in the back of the head or neck and accompanied by giddiness, seeing double, fortification figures, ataxia or slurred speech.

Meningitis

In meningitis headache is associated with fever and stiffness of the neck and sometimes with vomiting and photophobia (dislike of light). In an old person a meningitis can cause confusion with little or no headache.

Trauma to brain

Headache is likely after concussion as part of the post-concussional syndrome. It can be present on recovery from concussion or start later. Other features of the post-concussional syndrome are fatigue, irritability, nervousness, anxiety, insominia, giddiness and over-sensitivity to noise.

Cranial arteritis

In this condition attacks of pain occur in the temporal, occipital and facial areas, and sometimes in other parts of the body. The pain is throbbing and severe to an agonizing degree. The temporal artery may be thickened and tender, and the skin over it reddened. Other features can be blurring or loss of vision and paralysis of the motor nerves of the eye. An attack is commonly preceded by several months of malaise, slight pyrexia, loss of weight and pain in muscles and joints.

Pyrexia

Headache is common in pyrexia from any cause. It can be severe in:

influenza,   meningitis,
smallpox,   typhoid fever,
Q fever.

Alcohol and drugs

Headache can occur after:

alcoholic excess,
some general anaesthetics,
barbiturates and other hypnotics,
oral contraceptives,
glyceryl trinitrate,
MAO tranquillisers if the patient takes food containing tyramine, which is present in meat extracts, cheese, yoghurt, broad beans and red wine.

5. Pain in the Face

Pain in the face can be due to dental, naso-pharyngeal, ophthalmic, neurological and other diseases. In neurological diseases the trigeminal (fifth cranial) nerve is the one involved because it supplies the face through its three branches—the ophthalmic nerve, the maxillary nerve and the **mandibular nerve**.

Causes of pain in the face

Dental disease
Maxillary and frontal sinusitis
Diseases of the parotid gland
Diseases of the eye
Herpes zoster
Post-herpetic neuralgia
Trigeminal neuralgia
Glossopharyngeal neuralgia
Temperomandibular neuralgia
Atypical neuralgia
Studer's neuralgia
Raeder's neuralgia
Costen's syndrome
Osteomyelitis
Carcinoma of maxilla
Carcinoma of tongue

Dental disease

Dental caries and *dental abscesses* are common causes of pain in the face and jaws. The pain may be referred to the frontal and temporal regions of the head or to the ear.

Maxillary and frontal sinusitis

(a) *Maxillary sinusitis* causes pain in the cheek. The pain is often throbbing and made worse by moving the head, stooping, and walking. There will be a history of an upper respiratory tract infection or of a dental infection of the upper jaw or the extraction of a tooth from it. The cheek will be tender, and the patient will have a nasal discharge and a slight rise of temperature.

(b) *Frontal sinusitis* causes pain just above the eye. The pain is periodic, becoming worse during the morning and decreasing during the afternoon. There will be a history of an upper respiratory tract infection. The bone over the sinus will be tender on firm pressure.

Diseases of the eye

Pain in and around the eye can be caused by:

(a) an error of refraction,

(b) a corneal ulcer,

(c) iritis,

(d) acute glaucoma, in which increased intraocular pressure produces headache, impaired vision and seeing haloes or coloured rings.

Diseases of the parotid gland

(a) An *infection of the parotid gland* causes pain as the gland is enclosed within a capsule which is stretched by an inflammation. This happens in:

> *mumps*: at first in one gland, then in the other,
> *acute suppurative parotitis*: in one or both glands, as a complication of a severe illness,
> *chronic recurrent parotitis*: recurrent attacks of pain and swelling of both glands, usually in children.

(b) *Carcinoma of the parotid gland* produces a rapidly growing, hard, painful lump; the facial (seventh cranial) nerve can be invaded as it passes through the gland, with the production of facial paralysis on that side.

Herpes zoster

Severe pain, burning and itching in the skin supplied by one of the three branches of the trigeminal nerve are early features of herpes zoster and precede the rash by about 48 hours. The rash is an erythema with vesicles. The disease occurs in middle-aged or old people, and is due to infection of the ganglion of the trigeminal nerve by a reawakened chickenpox virus which has laid dormant in the tissues since an attack of chickenpox in childhood. If the ophthalmic nerve is involved, corneal ulceration can develop in the eye and threaten eyesight by producing scar tissue.

Post-herpetic neuralgia

This is a severe burning pain which can last for months or years after an attack of herpes zoster. The patient is usually old, and the area supplied by the ophthalmic nerve is the part usually involved. The pain can be continuous and intolerable and can make the patient acutely depressed.

Trigeminal neuralgia

In this condition bouts of pain occur in one or more of the areas supplied by the branches of the trigeminal nerve. The area supplied by the maxillary nerve is the one usually affected. Typically the pain is brought on by talking, eating, washing or shaving, and there are small 'trigger zones' in the face, stimulation of which sets off an attack. The pain occurs in bouts of brief attacks of severe electric-shock-like pain. Multiple bouts occur during a day; attacks do not usually happen at night. Bouts of pain tend to occur over weeks, and there may be periods of remission of up to two years. In addition to the bouts of pain, there may be a dull continuous ache. The patient is usually over the age of 60.

Glossopharyngeal neuralgia

In this condition paroxysms of intense pain, similar to those of trigeminal neuralgia, occur in the sensory distribution of the glossopharyngeal (ninth cranial) nerve. Pain is felt deep in the ear or in the fauces. Swallowing can set off an attack. The patient is usually middle-aged or old. It is much less common than trigeminal neuralgia.

Temperomandibular neuralgia

Attacks of pain occur in the ear and lower jaw. It is thought that it is due to malfunctioning of the temperomandibular joint due to loss of molar teeth. The patient is middle-aged or old.

Atypical neuralgia

This condition affects women only. It is a continuous burning pain which occurs in the cheek but can spread a little off the area supplied by the maxillary nerve. It can be precipitated by a dental extraction or a blow to the face, and lasts for months or years.

Studer's neuralgia

In this condition pain occurs in various parts of the face and radiates into the arm and hand.

Raeder's neuralgia

This is a severe pain in and around one eye. It is usually caused by malignant diseases of the base of the skull.

Costen's syndrome

This is a pain which shoots from the lower jaw up to the temporal region and is accompanied by various symptoms in the ear. It is thought to be due to dental malocclusion.

Osteomyelitis of jaw

Pain, swelling, trismus (clenching of the jaw), pyrexia and malaise are produced by osteomyelitis, infection of the bone arising as a complication of a dental extraction or a compound fracture. The lower jaw is more commonly affected than the upper.

Carcinoma of the maxilla

Pain in the cheek is a symptom of carcinoma of the maxilla. It can be associated with swelling of the cheek and with tears running down it owing to blocking of the nasolachrymal duct (through which tears should pass from the eye to the inside of the nose).

Carcinoma of the tongue

A carcinoma of the tongue is at first painless, but as it enlarges and spreads into the floor of the mouth and gums, it causes a pain, which radiates to the ear. The carcinoma appears as a lump, which ulcerates and bleeds.

6. Giddiness

Giddiness (vertigo) is a sensation of movement, with or without rotation, when no movement is taking place. People often say that they are giddy when they have some unsteadiness in standing or walking or feel 'light-headed' following a fever or prolonged immobilization in bed, with consequent hypotension, but these states are not real giddiness.

Giddiness is due to disease of the labyrinth of the inner ear or of the eighth cranial nerve which transmits sensations from it to the brain. It may be associated with deafness or nystagmus, a rhythmical oscillation of the eyeball, usually from side to side, sometimes up and down.

Causes of vertigo

Ménière's disease
multiple sclerosis
disease of the vertebral or basilar arteries
vestibular neuronitis
chronic ear disease
tumour of the eighth cranial nerve
positional vertigo
toxic effects of some drugs

Ménière's disease

Ménière's disease is characterized by attacks of severe, prostrating giddiness lasting for hours, deafness (which may be of one ear only), and severe tinnitus (ringing noises in the ear). The patient may complain of a feeling of fullness in the ear before an attack and of malaise and instability afterwards. He is likely to be under the age of fifty when attacks begin, and may have long periods of freedom from them.

Multiple sclerosis

Giddiness can be a feature of multiple (disseminated) sclerosis. It is likely to last for some weeks and then clear up. The patient is likely to give a history of other features of the disease, such as seeing double, having a temporary loss of sight, or having muscular weakness or sensory symptoms; and evidence of disease of the central nervous system is often found on examination. The attack of giddiness can, however, be the first evidence of the disease.

Disease of the vertebral or basilar arteries

The labyrinth of the inner ear is supplied with blood by a branch of the basilar artery; the basilar artery is formed by the union of the two vertebral arteries. Giddiness can be due to any obstruction to the supply of blood to the labyrinth. This obstruction can be due to atheroma of the vertebral or basilar arteries or to pressure by bony outgrowths on the vertebral arteries as they pass upwards through the holes in the lateral processes of the cervical vertebrae.

Vestibular neuronitis

This condition has been thought to be due to a virus infection of the labyrinth, but this has not been proved. The patient develops an attack of vertigo lasting for some hours or days, followed by a period of some weeks when he is liable to develop giddiness on changing suddenly the position of his head; after this he becomes free from attacks. He does not become deaf.

Chronic ear disease

Giddiness can be due to a spread of infection from a chronic otitis media. There is a history of pain in the ear, a discharge, and deafness in the ear.

Tumour of the eighth cranial nerve

A tumour of the eighth cranial nerve is likely to cause slight giddiness, deafness in the ear, and tinnitus.

Positional vertigo

The patient complains that he becomes giddy when he lies down in bed, turns over or get up; he may be able to lie only on one side. The condition can follow an ear infection or a head injury.

Toxic effects of some drugs

Streptomycin and kanamycin can damage the labyrinth and cause giddiness.

7. Confusion

Confusion is a state of impaired consciousness in which the patient is imperfectly aware of what is going on around him. He is muddled in his thoughts and can become deluded or hallucinated. *Disorientation* is a form of confusion in which there is a faulty appreciation of time, place or person, the patient not knowing what time of day it is, or where he is, or who he is. *Delirium* is a severe confusion in which the patient completely or nearly completely loses contact with reality.

Confusion is due to malfunctioning of cells in the cerebral cortex as a result of a raised temperature, electrolyte imbalance, disturbance of metabolism, lack of oxygen, abnormal electrical discharges in the brain or destruction of brain tissue.

Causes of confusion

Infections
Brain injury
Dementia
Cardiac, renal or hepatic failure
Endocrine abnormalities
Poisons and drugs
Extreme mental and physical exhaustion

Infections

An infection of the brain and meninges or any severe infection of the body can cause confusion. Confusion is likely in:

encephalitis
meningitis
pneumonia
typhoid fever, untreated, in 2nd–3rd week
typhus fever
Q fever

Brain injury

Confusion can be due to:

 concussion
 chronic subdural haematoma

(a) *Concussion.* Confusion is common after concussion. The longer the period of unconsciousness, the longer and worse will be the confusion.

(b) *Chronic subdural haematoma.* There should be a history of injury to the head, although the injury may have been slight. The patient is likely to have confusion, headache and drowsiness; he may be apathetic or excited. Typical of the condition is a daily variation in symptoms, the patient appearing seriously ill one day and much better the next.

Brain disease

Confusion can occur in several diseases of the brain, especially:

 epilepsy,
 multiple sclerosis,
 cerebral tumour,
 cerebral abscess.

(a) *Epilepsy.* Confusion can last for a short time after a fit; during it the patient may commit acts of which later he has no knowledge. In *temporal lobe epilepsy* confusion can be part of a syndrome in which occur peculiar dream states, peculiar sensations, movements of the tongue and lips, restlessness and sometimes violence.

(b) *Multiple (disseminated) sclerosis.* Patients can have acute attacks of confusion from which they recover, but after which they may show a further deterioration in their physical condition.

(c) *Cerebral tumour or abscess* causes confusion by increasing the intracranial pressure or locally damaging the brain.

Dementia

Confusion can be a symptom of any dementia:

 senile dementia,

arteriosclerotic dementia,
presenile dementia.

(a) *Senile dementia.* Acute confusional states can occur in which the patient becomes confused, noisy, disorientated and restless. He will be showing a progressive deterioration with a decline of intelligence, memory loss, emotional liability, speech difficulties and a decline in physical health. He will be over the age of 60.

(b) *Arteriosclerotic dementia.* In this condition acute confusional states similar to those that occur in senile dementia can occur; but the deterioration in this condition is intermittent with deterioration following each exacerbation of the disease and some temporary improvement between the actute phases. The patient will be over 50.

(c) *Presenile dementia.* In this condition, of which there are several types, the confusion and decline are similar to those in senile dementia, but the patient is younger, usually between 40 and 60.

Cardiac, renal and hepatic failure

Confusion is due in these conditions to impaired oxygenation of the blood or biochemical abnormalities which interfere with the correct functioning of cerebral cells.

(a) *Cardiac failure.* There can be delirium, auditory and visual hallucinations, disorientation in time and place, and terror. The patient is likely to be cyanosed and have dyspnoea; his liver may be enlarged and tender and he may have ascites and oedema. He will show evidence of the disease which has caused the heart to fail.

(b) *Renal failure* (uraemia). Confusion is likely to be associated with gastro-intestinal disturbances, muscular weakness, cramps, hypertension, anaemia, purpura and bleeding from mucous membranes.

(c) *Hepatic failure.* Confusion can occur before the patient goes into coma. Confusion will be associated with slurred speech, increased salivation, increased muscle tone, a sweetish odour in the breath, and a 'hepatic flap' of the outstretched hands.

Endocrine abnormalities

(a) *Hyperthyroidism* (thyrotoxicosis). Acute thyroid crises can occur in this condition, the patient having confusion, delirium, a very rapid pulse, a raised temperature and diarrhoea. He can pass into coma. He is likely to have an enlarged thyroid gland, prominent eyes, tremor and anxiety.

(b) *Hypothyroidism* (myxoedema). Attacks of confusion, hallucinations and disturbed behaviour can occur in this condition. The patient is likely to be over 30 and to show obesity, dullness, constipation, muscular aching, a bloated face and swollen legs, a slow pulse and a low temperature.

(c) *Hypoglycaemia.* In this condition the blood sugar is abnormally low as a result of starvation, an overdose of insulin or a tumour of the islet cells of the pancreas. Confusion is associated with sweating, drowsiness, muscular twitching and sometimes fits; the patient can pass into coma. The condition will be quickly relieved by the administration of sugar.

(d) *Acute adrenal insufficiency* (adrenal crisis). This is due to an acute failure of secretion of hormones from the cortex of the adrenal gland. Confusion is associated with weakness, apathy, cyanosed extremities and a fall in blood pressure (BP). Vomiting and diarrhoea can cause dehydration. The patient can pass into coma.

Poisons and drugs

Confusion can be due to:

>   alcohol,
>   barbiturate drugs,
>   LSD and other drugs of addiction,
>   chronic lead poisoning.

(a) *Alcohol.* Drunkenness is an acute confusional state due to an excessive consumption of alcohol. The person is likely to be confused, have slurred speech, stagger, behave irresponsibly, and smell of alcohol.

(b) *Barbiturates.* Overdosage with barbiturates and other hypnotics causes confusion, drowsiness and slurred speech.

(c) *LSD and other drugs of addiction.* A drug addict is likely to become confused and show other evidence of addiction: emaciation, septic sites of injection, irresponsible behaviour.

(d) *Chronic lead poisoning.* This can occur as an industrial disease. Confusion can be associated with abdominal pain, constipation or diarrhoea, headache, insomnia, fits or paralysis.

Extreme mental and physical exhaustion

Confusion can be caused by extreme stress, torture, danger of death, prolonged battle. The patient can develop an acute illness with confusion, disorientation, incoherent speech, delusions, hallucinations, anxiety, terror, a rapid pulse and tremor of lips and hands.

8. Coma

Consciousness is dependent upon the correct functioning of the cerebral hemispheres and of the reticular formation in the brain-stem. *Coma* is due to severe interference with the functioning of these structures, and in it the patient cannot be roused by stimuli, such as shouts and pricks. Milder degrees of interference cause clouding of consciousness from which the patient can be aroused by stimulation.

The causes of coma can be:

lesions within the skull,
general conditions affecting the brain.

When the cause is within the skull there is likely to be evidence of focal (i.e. local) damage to the drain, such as unequalness of pupil size, abnormalities in the response of the pupil to light and darkness, and signs of paralysis.

In some cases there may be more than one cause for coma: e.g. a drunk man may fall and receive a brain injury.

Lesions within the skull

Cerebral infarction
Cerebral haemorrhage
Extradural haematoma
Subdural haematoma
Subarachnoid haemorrhage
Brain injury
Epilepsy
Brain tumour
Meningitis and encephalitis

Cerebral infarction

Coma can be caused by a cerebral infarction due to the blocking of a cerebral artery by a clot of blood, etc. Whether or

31

not coma is produced depends upon the size of the infarction, the part of the brain involved, and the steepness of the rise of intracranial pressure which follows. In the common form of stroke the infarction involves a large part of the cerebral hemisphere, the rise in pressure is steep and coma profound. With infarction of the brainstem (midbrain, pons and medulla oblongata) coma can occur quickly. Evidence of focal involvement will be found according to the part of the brain involved.

Cerebral haemorrhage

The site of a cerebral haemorrhage is usually in one cerebral hemisphere. The patient is usually old and there may be a history of previous infarctions. The patient may complain of headache or vomit before he collapses and passes into coma. He is likely to show a hemiparesis. Breathing is deep and sterterous; there may be Cheyne-Strokes breathing; the pulse is full; the pupils are fixed and dilated; fits may occur.

Extradural haematoma

Coma can occur as a result of bleeding between the skull and dura mater. A clot of blood forms and the intracranial pressure rises.

Subdural haematoma

Injury to the head can cause bleeding between the dura mater and the brain with the production of a clot of blood which presses on the brain. Symptoms may not occur for days, weeks or months after the injury, which may have been slight. Before the onset of drowsiness, the patient complains of severe headache. A distinguishing feature of this kind of haemorrhage is that there may be day to day variations in the degree of drowsiness or unconsciousness, with the patient being seriously affected one day and apparently normal the next.

Subarachnoid haemorrhage

Blood in the subarachnoid space can be due to bleeding from a berry aneurysm on the circle of Willis or to injury. The patient usually has time to complain of an intense headache before losing consciousness. The neck is usually stiff; tendon jerks are at first abolished, and the plantar responses are extensor.

Brain injury

Concussion after head injury is common. There is immediate loss of consciousness with paralysis of voluntary muscles. The state of unconsciousness can last from seconds to many days, and on emerging from any prolonged concussion the patient is likely to pass through a period of drowsiness and confusion and have a headache. In very severe cases the patient dies in coma.

Epilepsy

Unconsciousness after a fit does not usually last for more than 30 minutes. The patient may have been incontinent or urine or have bitten himself. He may have sustained a head injury if he fell to the ground, and in severe epilepsy his face and scalp may be scarred by old injuries. Hypertrophy of the gums can often be observed in patients who have been taking phenytoin. (See Section 11.)

Brain tumour

With a brain tumour coma is due to the increasing intracranial pressure and displacement of the intracranial contents. It is likely to be severe if the rate is rapid as can occur when a tumour is rapidly expanded by a haemorrhage into it. Other clinical features that are likely to have occurred are: increasing headache, vomiting, double vision, fits, drowsiness, and any focal features due to the precise position of the tumour in or on the outside of the brain.

Meningitis and encephalitis

Consciousness is commonly impaired in all forms of meningitis and encephalitis. Other features likely to be present are fever, headache, vomiting, cerebral irritation, head retraction, fits, and paralysis of cranial nerves.

General conditions causing coma

Alcoholic poisoning
Drug overdose
Diabetic crisis
Hypoglycaemia
Hypothermia
Hypothyroidism
Respiratory, cardiac, renal and hepatic failure
Hypertensive encephalopathy
Cerebral malaria
Carbon monoxide poisoning

Alcoholic poisoning

In unconsciousness due to alcoholic poisoning a history of drinking may be obtained. The patient may have gone through a period of confusion, slurred speech, unsteady gait and disturbed behaviour. Coma can come on quickly. The patient is likely to smell of drink. He is at first pale and flaccid; as the coma deepens, breathing becomes sterterous and the pulse bounding; later the breathing becomes shallow and the pulse weak, and the BP falls.

Drug overdose

A drug overdose may be an accident, a suicidal attempt, or taken by an addict. Drugs which cause unconsciousness in overdoses include:

antihistamines
barbiturates and other hypnotics
bromides
morphine and other opium derivatives
pethidine
antidepressants

Coma is due to the depressant action of the drug on the central nervous system. Respiration is slow and sterterous or rapid and shallow. Muscle tone is reduced. Tendon reflexes are weak or absent. Retention of urine can occur.

Diabetic coma

That the patient is a diabetic may be known or he may carry a card saying so. There is a history of a slow onset—over days—and a development from confusion through drowsiness into coma. The patient's breath will smell of new-mown hay due to the excretion of ketones through the lungs. Respiration is slow and deep, the pulse is weak, the BP is low, and the skin is dry. Sugar and ketones are found in the urine, and the blood sugar is high.

Hypoglycaemia

A hypoglycaemic coma (i.e. one due to too low a blood sugar) differs from a diabetic coma in that it comes on quickly, the patient's breath does not smell of new-mown hay, he has a normal or raised BP and rapid shallow respirations, and he sweats profusely. He may have muscular twitchings or a fit. Hemiparesis (a paralysis of one side) may occur, to disappear with successful treatment.

Hypothermia

The weather will be very cold and the patient an old man or woman too poor to be able to afford adequate heating. The body is very cold, the deep body temperature being found to be below 35°C (95°F) when recorded on a special low-temperature thermometer kept in the rectum for 5 minutes. The face is puffy, the pulse-rate slow, BP low, and respiration slow and shallow.

Hypothyroidism

'A myxoedemic coma' can occur in severe hypothroidism, usually when the weather is very cold. The patient is likely to have a dry, coarse skin, a bloated face, loss of hair from the scalp and eyebrows, myxoedematous limbs, a slow pulse and a low temperature. Bruising, bleeding from the gastro-intestinal tract and cerebral haemorrhage can occur as a result of an increased permeability of the capillaries.

Respiratory, cardiac, renal and hepatic failure

Evidence of severe respiratory, cardiac renal or hepatic failure is present. A period of delirium usually precedes unconsciousness. Muscular twitching and tremors can occur.

Hypertensive encephalopathy

Hypertensive encephalopathy is a crisis which can occur in any kind of hypertension and is due to the effects on the brain of a sudden rise in a BP which is already high. Previous evidence of hypertension is usually available, and there may be a history of previous attacks. The crisis begins with a headache, and vomiting, after which there may be a period of impaired unconsciousness. Recovery usually occurs within a few hours or days.

Cerebral malaria

'Cerebral malaria' can occur in a severe malarial infection by *P. falciparum.* The patient has usually been ill for a long time, but the condition can occur suddenly in a first attack of the disease. The patient has a remittent temperature, passes through drowsiness into coma, may develop muscular twitching and fits, and may be incontinent of urine and faeces.

Carbon monoxide poisoning

The skin is pink when exposure to carbon monoxide has been sudden, when the blood is highly saturated with the gas, and when the patient is not anaemic. With gradual exposure to carbon monoxide, as can happen in some industrial accidents, the skin is grey and the lips flaked with foam. The respiration is rapid and shallow, and Cheyne-Stokes breathing can occur.

9. Loss of Memory

Loss of memory (amnesia) can be for recent events, for distant events, or global (total) for both recent and remote events.

Loss of memory

Brain injury
Cerebral tumour
Dementia
Alcoholism
Hysteria

Brain injury

Loss of memory can be due to a single blow to the head, to multiple blows, or to ECT (electrocerebral therapy).

(a) *Post-concussional syndrome.* On recovery from concussion a patient may show:

> retrograde amnesia,
> post-traumatic amnesia.

(i) *Retrograde amnesia* is a loss of memory in which the patient is unable to remember the blow which knocked him out and events for a variable time before it. After a short period of concussion, the retrograde amnesia may be only for a few seconds, but after prolonged concussion it may be for weeks, months or years. A patient may have 'islands of memory', i.e. he can remember individual events in an otherwise forgotten past.

(ii) *Post-traumatic amnesia* is a loss of memory from the time of the injury until the patient becomes continuously aware of his surroundings, which comes after a period of being intermittently aware of them.

(b) *Punch drunkenness.* Loss of memory is a feature of punch drunkenness in a boxer who has been knocked out several times and is due to cerebral deterioration following blows to the head and banging his head on the floor of the ring when he falls. Amnesia is likely to be associated with mental slowness, slurred speech, ataxia, a coarse tremor of the outstretched hands, fatuousness, and outbursts of rage, jealousy and violence. The patient may have cataracts (opacities in the lens) due to blows to the eye.

(c) *ECT* (electrocerebral therapy). A patient who has had ECT is liable to develop loss of memory as a result of the death of cerebral nerve cells due to the passage of an electrical current through the brain. The more times he has ECT the worse is his loss of memory likely to be. It may be lost indefinitely and be associated with impairment of concentration.

Cerebral tumour

Loss of memory can be an early symptom of a cerebral tumour. When the tumour is in the frontal lobe, it is likely to be associated with apathy, poverty of ideas, facetiousness and incontinence. Headache and vomiting are liking to ensue.

Dementia

Loss of memory is a feature of all dementias. It can occur in:
> senile dementia,
> presenile dementia,
> arterio-sclerotic dementia,
> dementia due to head-injury,
> dementia due to progressive disease of the brain: paralysis agitans, multiple (disseminated) sclerosis, Huntington's chorea, general paralysis of the insane, etc.

Usually the loss of memory is for recent events, but in time and with the further progress of the disease, it becomes global.

Alcoholism

(a) *Chronic alcoholism.* Loss of memory, carelessness, irresponsibility, emotional liability, paranoid ideas, and outbursts of violence occur as features of chronic alcoholism, are are likely to be associated with physical disease due to alcoholism: obesity, chronic bronchitis, chronic gastritis, cirrhosis of the liver, cardiovascular degeneration and peripheral neuritis.

(b) *Korsakov's syndrome.* This form of cerebral degeneration is due to chronic alcoholism and is characterized by (a) a profound and in the end global loss of memory, (b) confabulation —the patient tells wholly imaginary stories of what he has been doing.

Hysteria

Loss of memory can be one of the 'dissociative reactions' of hysteria, which can occur as a form of escape from a difficult situation. The patient reacts by losing his memory, completely or partially. He is likely to have shown other signs of hysteria. A *fugue state* is a twilight state in which the patient wanders about, his memory impaired and often disorientated in time, place and person.

10. Anxiety

Anxiety is a normal response to stress. Faced with a difficult situation any normal person can become nervous, tense, worried, tremulous, have a rapid heart rate, be unable to concentrate, develop a stammer or tremor, or be unable to sleep soundly. The amount of stress that can bring on anxiety varies from person to person. Anxiety is abnormal when it is brought on by little or no stress, is severe, or continues after the cause of the stress is removed or disappears.

Causes of anxiety

Anxiety state
Hyperthyroidism
Excessive coffee drinking
Depression
Delirium tremens
Post-concussional syndrome
Hypoglycaemia
Temporal lobe epilepsy
Phaeochromocytoma

Anxiety state

An anxiety state can occur at any age and in variable degrees of severity.

In an *acute anxiety state* brought on by severe stress the patient is tense sometimes to the point of immobilization, his heart rate and respiratory rates are increased, his pupils are dilated, and he sweats profusely. He is likely to have insomnia or if he sleeps to have terrifying dreams.

In a *chronic anxiety state* the degree of anxiety can vary from day to day, or week to week but never completely disappears. Among the various things the patient may complain of are nervousness, palpitations, fatigue, loss of appetite, fainting, blackouts, giddiness, sweating, tremulousness, stammering, frequency of micturition, diarrhoea or constipation, and fears of death or going insane.

A *phobic state* is an anxiety state with a specific fear, e.g. *claustrophobia*: a fear of being shut up and so of any enclosed space; *agoraphobia*: a fear of open spaces, streets, fields.

An *effort syndrome* is an acute anxiety state with emphasis on the circulatory system. The patient is usually of asthenic build and in face of hard physical work, such as military training, develops palpitations, irregular cardiac action,precordial pain, shortness of breath and excessive fatigue.

Hyperthyroidism (thyrotoxicosis)

Anxiety is a common feature of hyperthyroidism, in which condition excessive amounts of thyroid hormones are secreted into the blood. The degree of illness varies from mild to severe, and the onset from insidious to rapid. The patient is likely to be anxious, irritable, distractible and restless, and will have poor sleep disturbed by anxiety dreams. The thyroid gland is usually noticeably larger and firmer than normal. The eyes are prominent. The patient has a fine tremor of fingers and tongue. The heart rate is increased, and artrial fibrillation and heart failure can develop. The appetite remains good, but weight is lost in spite of this.

Excessive coffee drinking

Anxiety, nervousness, rapid or irregular heart rate, tremulousness, headache and insomnia can be produced by excessive coffee drinking, the subject thus consuming large amounts of caffeine, and disappear when the coffee drinking is stopped or sharply reduced.

Depression

Anxiety is a feature of some depressive illness (indeed an anxiety state is regarded by many psychiatrists as a form of depression). Anxiety is particularly likely to be a prominent feature of depressive illness occurring in the second half of life, with the patient becoming anxious, tense, pacing up and down, and preoccupied with depressive ideas and thoughts of suicide.

Delirium tremens

Anxiety is an early symptom of delirium tremens, which is a toxic-confusional state brought on by chronic alcoholism and precipitated by a particularly long bout of heavy drinking or by an accident or an illness. In addition to anxiety the patient is in the early stages likely to have broken sleep, irritability, and bad temper from which he passes into confusion and restlessness with attacks of terror and sometimes fits. He can develop pneumonia or sustain a fracture by falling out of bed.

Post-concussional syndrome

After a severe concussion the patient is likely to pass through a post-concussional state characterized by anxiety, headache, insomnia, giddiness, irritability, difficulty in concentrating or blackouts. The degree of severity of the symptoms, including anxiety, depends upon the length of the concussion, the personality of the patient, and the incentives he has to recover or remain disabled.

Hypoglycaemia

Anxiety, sweating, flushing, a rapid heart rate and giggling can occur with a mild degree of hypoglycaemia (a lowering of the blood sugar below normal) and confusion, coma and fits with a severe degree. The hypoglycaemia can be due to:

(a) an overdose of insulin or not taking enough sugar to cover a dose of it;

(b) an islet cell tumour of the pancreas which secretes an excessive amount of insulin;

(c) after a partial gastrectomy, when after a meal the blood sugar first rises sharply as a result of rapid absorption in the small intestine and then falls and produces hypoglycaemia.

Temporal lobe epilepsy

Attacks of anxiety recurring episodically can be a sign of

temporal lobe epilepsy. This form of epilepsy is characterized by peculiar mental states, which can be varied in content, anxiety, feelings of strangeness, smacking of the lips or tongue, impulsive behaviour or violence. An EEG may show abnormal discharges from one or both temporal lobes of the brain.

Phaeochromocytoma

This is an uncommon tumour of the adrenal medulla which secretes excessive amounts of adrenaline or nor-adrenaline. As a result the patient has attacks, usually lasting 10–15 minutes, sometimes longer, in which he is anxious, sweats profusely, has palpitations, irregular heart action, pallor, coldness, pounding in the head, nausea and vomiting. Most patients with it have hypertension. Attacks may occur spontaneously or be brought on by exertion, emotion, palpitation of the abdomen and minor operations.

11. Fits

A *fit* is the result of a disorder of brain function in which there is an excessive synchronous discharge by a group of nerve-cells and the spread of this discharge along paths determined by its point of origin and the anatomical arrangements of associated nerve fibres. The precipitating factor can be:

(a) a cerebral abnormality

(b) a general condition of the body affecting cerebral function.

Idiopathic epilepsy is epilepsy for which no cause can be found; other names for it are cryptogenic and constitutional epilepsy.

1. CEREBRAL ABNORMALITIES

Causes of epilepsy: cerebral abnormalities

Congenital abnormality of cerebral development
Birth injury or anoxia
Injury to brain
Encephalitis, meningitis
Syphilis of brain
Cerebral tumour
Cerebral abscess
Dementia
Cysticercosis

Congenital abnormality of cerebral development

Epilepsy of any kind is a common occurrence when the cerebral hemispheres have not developed normally (fibrosis of brain, cysts, hydrocephalus, etc.). It is commonly associated with:

44

spasticity,
involuntary movements,
mental retardation,
defect of sight or hearing.

Birth injury or anoxia

Fits may be due to cerebral injury and haemorrhages or anoxia during birth. It is not easy sometimes to distinguish whether fits in an infant are due to these or to some congenital abnormality of the brain.

Injury to brain

Major fits, and sometimes other kinds, occur in 2–4 per cent of brain injuries. They usually begin within 2 years of the injury; fits occurring within a few days usually stop spontaneously, and the longer the interval between the injury and the onset of epilepsy the more likely are fits to persist.

Encephalitis, meningitis

Fits can be produced by any encephalitis or meningitis. Other likely features are fever, headache, vomiting, confusion, a stiff neck and cranial nerve paralysis.

Syphilis of the brain

(a) *Meningovascular syphilis.* Fits can occur in meningovascular syphilis, which appears within a few months of the primary syphilitic infection or not until several years later. Other features vary; they include headache, impairment of memory and intelligence, aphasia, hemiplegia, and cranial nerve paralysis.

(b) *General paralysis of the insane* (GPI). A fit can be the first sign (as well as occurring later) of this tertiary syphilitic disease of the brain. Untreated, the patient develops a progressive dementia, paralysis, tremor, slurred speech, and incontinence. The disease develops 5–25 years after the primary syphilitic infection, and the patient is usually 30–50 years old. The occurrence of a fit for the first time in a patient of this age group would suggest that he had either general paralysis of the insane or a cerebral tumour.

Cerebral tumour

A fit is commonly an early feature of a cerebral tumour and sometimes precedes other symptoms by months or years. It can be a general or a focal fit. Signs of raised intracranial pressure (headache, vomiting, drowsiness, coma, papilloedema) eventually appear and there may be other localization signs which indicate the position of the tumour in the brain.

Cerebral abscess

Fits, general or focal, can be produced by a cerebral abscess. The abscess will be secondary to either a septic focus in the head (chronic otitis media, nasal infection, carbuncle, etc.) or to a septic focus in the chest (lung abscess, bronchiectasis, empyema). The patient will have a raised temperature and is likely to show signs of intracranial pressure (headache, vomiting drowsiness, coma, papilloedema), and there may be localized signs which indicate the position of the abscess in the brain.

Dementia

Fits can occur in any degenerative condition of the brain: senile dementia, presenile dementia, arteriosclerotic dementia, dementia due to any other chronic brain disease.

Cysticercosis

Focal epilepsy can occur in this condition in which cysts form in the brain following ingestion of eggs of the tapeworm *T. solium*. The cysts in time become calcified and are then visible on an X-ray.

2. GENERAL CONDITIONS

Certain general conditions of the body can produce epilepsy by interfering with metabolic process in the brain and with its functioning.

Causes of epilepsy: general conditions

In infancy: dentition, fever, gastro-intestinal infec-
tions, rickets, acute allergic reactions, breath-
holding
Heart block
Hypertensive encephalopathy
Hypoglycaemia
Eclampsia
Lead poisoning
Carbon monoxide poisoning

In infancy: dentition, fever, gastro-intestinal infections, rickets, acute allergic reactions

In all these conditions some infants can have fits, possibly because of some metabolic instability or some minor, and otherwise undetectable, brain damage. Multiple or prolonged fits can further damage the brain and produce still more fits.

Heart block

A fit can occur with prolonged heart-block (See Stokes-Adam syndrome).

Hypertensive encephalopathy

Fits, general or focal, can occur during an attack of hypertensive encephalopathy. Such an attack is due to a still higher rise of BP in a patient who already has hypertension. An attack lasts for hours or days, and in it the patient is likely to have intense headache, drowsiness or vomiting, and sometimes hemiparesis and fits.

Hypoglycaemia

A generalized fit can occur if hypoglycaemia is so severe as to produce coma. Hypoglycaemia (a reduction of the blood sugar below the normal level) can be due to (a) an overdose of insulin, (b) not taking enough carbohydrate to cover a normal dose of insulin, or (c) a tumour of the islets of Langerhans, which produces an excessive amount of insulin. A mild degree of hypoglycaemia will produce sweating, tremor, a rapid pulse and emotional liability; a severe degree will produce confusion, coma and fits.

Renal failure

Generalized fits can occur in uraemia produced by renal failure. They can be precipitated by fluid retention or a blood transfusion, or occur as a symptom of hypertensive encephalopathy. There will be a history of renal disease and other evidence of renal failure: gastro-intestinal disturbances, tremor, muscular twitching, hypertension, anaemia, heart failure, a decreased excretion of urine, albuminuria.

Eclampsia

Generalized fits are the essential feature of eclampsia, a toxaemia of pregnancy. They are preceded by albuminuria, hypertension, frontal headache, vomiting, pain over an enlarged liver, and flashes or spots of light in front of the eyes.

Lead poisoning

General fits can be a feature of lead poisoning. A fit can be the first feature and cause a diagnosis of cerebral tumour to be provisionally made. Other evidence of lead poisoning is: headache, irritability, insomnia, confusion, tremor, paralysis and attacks of abdominal colic.

Carbon monoxide poisoning

Fits can occur in carbon monoxide poisoning as a result of anoxia of the brain.

3. CLINICAL VARIETIES OF EPILEPSY

Epileptic fits are classified clinically into several varieties. The variation is due to the different places in the brain in which a fit can arise and their nervous connections, and to the cause of the fit.

Clinical varieties of epilepsy

Major fit
Minor fit
Temporal lobe epilepsy
Focal fit
Inhibitory (akinetic) epilepsy
Myoclonic epilepsy
Autonomic epilepsy
Reflex epilepsy
Status epilepticus

Major fit (grand mal). A major fit is unmistakable. The patient loses consciousness, sometimes after a preliminary warning called an aura; develops a tonic stiffening of his muscles, cyanosis and sterterous breathing; then develops clonic jerking of the muscles, which violent at first become gradually less violent; and then passes into a state of flaccidity with mental confusion for a few minutes. Complications are: incontinence of urine, biting the tongue, dislocation of a joint, fracture of a bone, injuries due to falling, aggressive behaviour (epileptic furor) during the period of confusion following the fit. Death can occur in a fit.

Minor fit (petit mal). A minor fit occurring singly, can be difficult to detect. The patient has a sudden short period of loss of attention (an 'absence'), with arrest of movement and speech, and sometimes with flickering of the eyes, pallor or flushing. Frequent attacks can occur.

Temporal lobe epilepsy (psychomotor epilepsy). Features of this kind of epilepsy vary and diagnosis is often difficult. The patient may become confused and unaware or only partly aware of his surroundings, wander about, act aggressively, have champing movements of his jaw, etc., with a complete amnesia for the attack. A major fit occurs sooner or later.

Focal fit (Jacksonian epilepsy). This variety usually begins with muscle twitching in the hand and spreads up the arm, into the face or down the leg on the same side. Abnormal sensations can spread in the same way.

Inhibitory (akinetic) epilepsy. In this variety the patient suffers a sudden loss of consciousness with loss of muscular power and slumps to the floor. An attack lasts for a few seconds and full consciousness is quickly recovered, unless the patient has suffered concussion when his head hits the ground.

Myoclonic epilepsy. Sudden, brief, local or general muscular jerks occur. There is no loss of consciousness unless it leads up to a major fit.

Myoclonic jerking occurring when a person is falling asleep is not to be regarded as abnormal and is not of any importance.

Autonomic epilepsy (vasovagal attacks). Attacks of epigastric pain with a rapid and sometimes irregular pulse, low BP, sweating, cold hands and feet, and a feeling of impending death, last for 10–30 minutes and end suddenly.

Reflex epilepsy. These are attacks of epilepsy (usually major or focal fits) produced by some definite sensory stimulus, such as a flickering light, a tune, a particular noise, etc..

Status epilepticus. This is the continuous recurrence of an epileptic fit. It can occur with major fits, minor fits, focal fits, myoclonic fits and temporal lobe epilepsy. It can last for hours or days. Complications: heart failure, respiratory infection.

12. Involuntary Movements

Involuntary movements are movements made without a person wishing to make them; they are often uncontrollable.

Principle types

Tremor
Tic
Chorea
Myoclonus
Athetoid movement

---

1. TREMOR

Tremor is a rhythmically recurring slight movement.

Common tremors

Physiological tremor
Pathological tremors: tremor of
   paralysis agitans
   parkinsonism
   thyrotoxicosis
   cerebellar disease
   anxiety state

(a) Physiological tremor

This is a normal postural tremor of the outstretched fingers which occurs in all people in varying degrees. A postural tremor is one which is most obvious on maintaining a posture. It is made worse by anxiety, coffee and alcohol.

(b) Paralysis agitans

Tremor is one of the characteristic features of paralysis agitans (Parkinson's disease), which is due to a degeneration of the basal ganglia of the brain. The other characteristic features are poverty of movement and rigidity. The patient is likely to be over the age of fifty and the condition is likely to be diagnosed at sight, with the patient showing immobility of features, poverty of gestures, a slightly bowed posture and shuffling steps. The tremor usually involves the muscles of the forearm, hand and feet. It usually begins on one side of the body, affecting both limbs on that side before appearing on the other. It is fine and rapid, occurs at rest, and stops temporarily on voluntary movement of the part. It is made worse by fatigue, excitement and anxiety.

(c) Parkinsonism

A condition clinically similar to that of paralysis agitans and with the same kind of tremor can be due to:

> cerebral arteriosclerosis,
> other degenerative diseases of the brain,
> infections of the brain,
> certain drugs, especially phenothiazine drugs used as tranquillizers.

(d) Hyperthyroidism

A fine rapid tremor is present in hyperthyroidism (thyrotoxicosis). Other features likely to be present are: an enlarged thyroid gland, prominent staring eyes, dilated pupils, a rapid pulse, and sweating.

(e) Cerebellar diseases

The tremor due to cerebellar diseases is an intention tremor, i.e. a tremor which occurs on voluntary movements. Clinically it is demonstrated by asking the patient to touch his nose with his outstretched finger or to put one heel on the opposite knee and run it down the shin. It can interfere with any movements the patient wants to make, so that he has difficuly in feeding himself, dressing and undressing, picking up things, and walking.

The cerebellum is the part of the brain responsible for the coordination of muscular actions. The commonest cause of the tremor is multiple (disseminated) sclerosis. Other causes are atheroma of the vertebral, basilar or cerebellar arteries (which causes a reduction in the amount of blood supplied to the cerebellum) and a tumour of the cerebellum.

(f) Anxiety state

A fine rapid tremor is likely to be present in an anxiety state.

2. TIC

Tics are short muscular contractions which are repeated in the same muscles. They occur in about a quarter of normal children and nearly always disappear before adolescence; in a few people they persist throughout adult life. They usually produce blinking, lip-smacking, sniffing and shrugging the shoulders. They can sometimes be controlled by the patient, but the effort he makes may increase the anxiety he feels about them.

3. CHOREA

Chorea is a series of continuous, irregular muscular jerks, occurring in any group of voluntary muscles. The contractions, irregular in time and strength of contraction, interfere with normal movements and speech, prevent the patient from maintaining a steady grip, and cause him to lurch and stop and start when walking.

Main types of chorea

Rheumatic chorea
Huntington's chorea

(a) Rheumatic chorea

Rheumatic (Sydenham's) chorea is part of the rheumatic fever complex, occurring either on its own or in association with carditis, arthritis, and other signs of rheumatic fever. The patient is a child or occasionally a young pregnant woman. The usual complaints are that the child is dropping things, making faces at people, and cannot sit still. Handwriting deteriorates and speech may be jerky or unintelligible. The chorea usually lasts for several months and repeated attacks can occur.

(b) Huntington's chorea

Huntington's chorea is an inherited degenerative disease of the brain characterized by chorea and dementia. Either may occur first and both get progressively worse until the patient dies. The patient is usually over the age of thirty when symptoms appear. If the family history is known the diagnosis is easy to make; but when it is not, the diagnosis is not easy until both of the main features, the chorea and the dementia, are present. As the disease gets worse the muscular movements become greater and can keep the patient in a state of continuous movement.

4. MYOCLONUS

Myoclonus is a series of brief muscular twitches, which can occur regularly or irregularly in the same muscle group. It can occur:

> normally on falling asleep or waking up,
> as an epileptic phenomenon,
> in respiratory, renal or hepatic failure,
> in various degenerations and infections of the brain,
> as a withdrawal phenomenon in alcoholics and drug-
> addicts.

5. ATHETOID MOVEMENT

Athetoid movements are slow, irregular movements involving several muscle groups or the whole musculature. They are commonly seen in spastic patients and are likely to be associated with:

> spasticity of muscles,
> epilepsy,
> skeletal deformities,
> mental retardation.

The movements twist the limbs or body into abnormal positions and grossly interfere with normal movements. They are made worse by anxiety and excitement.

13. Difficulty in Speaking

Speaking is a complex activity in which many systems are co-ordinated. In medical use the term *speech* is used to describe writing, reading, hearing and speaking. The *speech centre* is situated in the left cerebral hemisphere in all right-handed people and probably in most left-handed people; it is situated in the lower parts of the frontal and parietal lobes and the upper part of the temporal lobe. It receives its blood supply through branches of the left middle cerebral artery. Difficulty in speaking may be due to faulty development of the brain, to psychogenic causes, to disease of the brain, to diseases of the larynx, and to intoxication by alcohol or drugs.

Difficulty in speaking

Developmental:	mental retardation
	congenital deafness
	delayed speech
Psychogenic:	stammering
	developmental mutism
	anxiety
	hysteria
Disease of brain:	congenital spasticity
	multiple sclerosis
	paralysis agitans
	disease of the speech centre
	myasthenia gravis
	pseudobulbar paralysis
	hepatolenticular degeneration
	delirium
	dementia
Disease of larynx:	laryngitis
	tumour of larynx
Intoxication:	alcohol
	drugs

DEVELOPMENTAL DIFFICULTIES

Mental retardation

Several retarded persons may not be able to speak at all or learn to speak a few words or simple sentences often with imperfect articulation owing to a failure of development of the cerebral hemispheres or disease of them.

Deafness

Congenitally deaf children or children with 'high tone deafness' (an inability to hear sounds above a certain frequency) do not learn to speak clearly or with normal inflection as they cannot hear words and cannot learn easily what sounds to make.

Delayed speech

Some children do not start to speak until they are 2–3 years old, but then start to speak well. There may be a familial incidence of late speaking. In *developmental mutism* speech is delayed until after 3 years in children who otherwise appear normal and is muddled and indistinct for several years; it is sometimes associated with left-handedness.

PSYCHOGENIC DIFFICULTIES

Stammering

Stammering is a defect of articulation with a sudden check in the utterance of words or a rapid repetition of the sound of a consonant. Spasmodic movements of the face and head may occur at the same time. It is precipitated by shyness, anxiety, self-consciousness and timidity, and may appear after a fright, an emotional strain or a severe illness. In some it is the result of a lesion in the speech centre of the brain.

Anxiety

Anxiety can cause stammering, the repetition of phrases or sentences, or a complete drying up of speech.

Hysteria

Mutism can be a feature of hysteria. The patient is not usually completely mute but speaks in a hoarse whisper.

DISEASES OF THE BRAIN

Congenital spasticity

A congenital spasticity of muscle due to imperfect development or congenital diseases of the brain interferes with speech by making articulation difficult. Involuntary movements add to the patient's difficulties. Speech can be bursts of incomprehensible sounds. The patient may have a good understanding of speech and knows what he wants to say, and the more desperate he becomes to express himself the worse becomes his articulation.

Multiple (disseminated) sclerosis

In the later stages of this disease speech can become 'scanning', i.e. syllables are separately pronounced.

Paralysis agitans

In this disease speech becomes monotonous and devoid of inflexion due to spasticity of the muscles of the larnyx, tongue and lips.

Disease of the speech centre of the brain

The speech centre of the brain can be damaged by an injury, pressed upon or invaded by a tumour, or have its blood supply diminished by disease of the arteries supplying it. Usually speech function as a whole is affected, but some parts of speech may be more affected than others: there may be impairment of spoken or written speech, or of the reception of speech, or a nominal aphasia (the patient is unable to name an object which he can recognize and of which he knows the function), or a jargon aphasia (the patient produces meaningless sounds).

Myasthenia gravis

Speech is likely to be impaired and become indistinct because of the abnormal fatigability of muscle which is the feature of this disease.

Progressive bulbar paralysis

This is one of the group of diseases called *motor neurone diseases*. They are characterized by muscle wasting and some spasticity. In this form the muscles to the larynx, tongue, pharynx and face waste. Speech is at first slurred and then a long moaning sound which the patient cannot control. At the same time swallowing becomes difficult, whistling and pursing the lips impossible, and the tongue is visibly wasted.

Hepatolenticular disease (Wilson's disease)

This disease of copper metabolism becomes manifest in child-hood. Due to disease of the brain speech becomes slurred, the face flattened and the limbs spastic. Cirrhosis of the liver produces jaundice and often an enlarged spleen. A greenish-brown ring of copper deposit may be visible in the eye at the corneo-sclerotic junction.

Delirium

Speech is impaired in any delirium. Against a background of impaired consciousness, dream state and hallucinations, speech is likely to be muttering and slurred with much repetition of phrases.

Dementia

Speech is progressively impaired in all dementias. With increasing intellectual deterioration, it becomes vague, irrele-vant, and in the end a babble of meaningless sounds.

Disease of the larynx

Hoarseness can be due to:
      laryngitis,

tuberculosis of the larynx,
a tumour, benign or malignant, of the larynx.

Intoxication

Speech becomes impaired and slurred in:

acute alcoholism,
overdosage of barbiturates and other sedatives or
hypnotics.

14. Difficulty in Walking

Difficulty in walking may be due to ill-fitting shoes, corns, arthritis, general weakness from any cause, or to diseases of the blood vessels supplying the legs, to diseases of muscle or to diseases of the nervous system.

1. DISEASES OF BLOOD VESSELS

Intermittent claudication

This is a painful cramp in the calf produced by walking and relieved by rest. It is liable to become progressively worse and reduces the distance a patient can walk. It can affect one or both legs. It is due to an inadequate blood supply to the calf muscles as a result of blocking of the femoral or popiteal arteries by atheroma, and is relieved by the establishment of an adequate collateral circulation. Gangrene of the toes develops if the blood supply to them is completely cut off.

Similar pain can occur in the muscles of the gluteal region or thigh by atheromatous blocking of the bifurcation of the aorta or of the iliac arteries.

2. DISEASE OF MUSCLE

Diseases of muscle

Pseudohypertrophic muscular dystrophy
Limb-girdle muscular dystrophy
Dystrophia myotonica
Tibialis anterior syndrome

Pseudohypertrophic muscular dystrophy

There are two types of this disease in which muscles become

61

enlarged before they waste. Both types interfere with walking.

(a) *Duchenne type.* This occurs in boys and is transmitted by women who are clinically normal. The calf muscles and deltoids are commonly affected early. The boy begins to have difficulty in walking and getting up off the floor by the age of 3, is usually unable to walk at all by 10, and dies before the age of 20 of a chest infection or heart failure.

(b) *Becker type.* This milder form of the disease begins later (5–25 years), runs a more chronic course, and is transmitted from affected males through carrier daughters to their grandsons. Walking becomes progressively more difficult, and the patient is likely to be confined to a wheelchair by middle age.

Limb-girdle muscular dystrophy

Walking is affected by wasting of the muscles of the pelvic girdle, which in some cases precedes wasting of the shoulder muscles. It begins at 10–20 years and patients are confined to a wheelchair by middle age.

Dystophia myotonica

Difficulty in walking and weakness of the hands are early features of this disease in which wasting occurs in many muscles and is associated with other abnormalities, including:

> cataracts in the eyes,
> frontal baldness in men,
> atrophy of testes or ovaries,
> cardiac muscle disease,
> mental abnormalities.

Tibialis anterior syndrome

Difficulty in walking and pain in front of one or both legs are due in this condition to swelling of the tibialis anterior muscle within its tough fibrous sheath.

3. DISEASES OF THE NERVOUS SYSTEM

Diseases of the nervous system

Congenital spastic paralysis
Poliomyelitis
Hemiplegia
Paralysis agitans
Parkinsonism
Multiple sclerosis
Disease of the cerebellum
Friedrich's ataxia
Tabes dorsalis
Peripheral neuropathy

Congenital spastic paralysis (cerebral diplegia)

This condition is due to either a failure of development of the brain or to degeneration of the brain as a result of prenatal conditions or brain damage during birth. Various degrees of spasticity, paralysis, contractures and involuntary movement can be present, and walking may be difficult or impossible. Some children with spasticity of the calf muscles walk on tip toe. Associated conditions are likely to be mental retardation and fits.

Poliomyelitis

In the paralytic form of this disease flaccid paralysis, loss of muscle tone and loss of reflexes are produced by damage of the anterior horn cells in the spinal cord. The legs are commonly affected. Following the acute attack various degrees of recovery can occur. Walking will be interfered with if some degree of paralysis persists in one or both legs. The paralysed muscles atrophy; an affected limb will not develop normally if the attack occurs before full growth has been achieved; and the limb is liable to become deformed by contractures and by the unopposed action of healthy muscles.

Hemiplegia

Paralysis of one side of the body (including the leg) will interfere with walking. Common causes are:

> injury to one side of the brain,
> multiple sclerosis,
> cerebral thrombosis or embolism,
> tumour of the brain.

After a stroke the patient may not be able to lift his foot off the ground and has to swing his leg round when trying to walk.

Paralysis agitans (Parkinson's disease)

In this condition the patient walks with short hurrying steps and without swinging his arms. He may not be able to stop himself from breaking into a shuffling run. It is a disease of the basal ganglia of the brain, of unknown causation, more common in men than women, and coming on at 45–65 years. Associated features are a stoop, a tremor of the hands at rest, a mask-like face and monotonous speech.

Parkinsonism

The clinical features of this condition are similar to those of paralysis agitans, and the patient develops the same walking difficulties. It has certain known causes and is not limited to older age groups. If caused by drugs the condition is reversible when they are stopped. Causes include:

> cerebral arteriosclerosis,
> certain drugs: phenothiazines, butyrophenones, rauwolfia alkaloids, tetrabenzene,
> poisoning by carbon monoxide, carbon disulphide, manganese,
> encephalitis lethargica.

Multiple (disseminated) sclerosis

Weakness in one or both legs is a common early symptom of this disease in which patches of degeneration appear in the central nervous system and nerve-fibres lose their myelin sheath. The onset of weakness in the legs can be so sudden that a man who has set off for a walk feeling perfectly well cannot manage to get home. Some patients develop a pattern in which fatigue and deterioration follow a period in which they walk normally. A hemiplegia is sometimes a sign of this disease.

Diseases of the cerebellum

Ataxia (incoordination of muscular action) is produced by disease of the cerebellum, in which muscular action is co-ordinated. The disease may be due to:

> inadequate blood supply due to atheroma of the vertebral or basilar arteries,
> multiple sclerosis,
> tumour,
> degeneration from unknown causes.

There can be various degrees of disability, from slight un-steadiness to complete inability to walk or stand. The gait is reeling and staggering, with the feet planted wide apart and brought down with a stamp. If the lesion in the cere-bellum is unilateral, there is a tendency to sway or deviate to the same side.

Friedreich's ataxia

A clumsy gait is an early sign of this disease, which is an inherited degeneration of the posterior columns of the spinal cord and of the cerebellum. The disease begins in childhood. The patient cannot co-ordinate his movements, he walks with unequal, irregular steps, plants his feet wide apart, and reels from side to side. The arms are also affected and speech becomes slurred.

Tabes dorsalis

In this condition the patient is unable to appreciate the exact position of his feet. He walks with them abnormally wide apart, tends to lift them too high, stamps them down hard, and eventually cannot walk without the aid of one or two sticks.

The disease is a tertiary syphilitic degeneration of the posterior columns of the spinal cord in which certain sensory impulses are conveyed to the brain. It begins at 30–45 years and is slowly progressive. Associated features are 'lightning pains', Argyll Robertson pupils (which react to accommodation, but not to light), loss of tendon reflexes, ulcers of the feet, enlarged joints, and visceral crises (acute painful disturbance of the stomach or other viscera).

Peripheral neuropathy

Difficulty in walking is a feature of peripheral neuropathy when the nerves to the legs are involved. The muscles become weak and waste; foot-drop can occur, and the patient lifts his legs up high to overcome it. Disturbances of sensation are likely. It can occur in:

diabetes mellitus,	chronic alcoholism,
beri-beri,	vitamin B_{12} deficiency,
uraemia,	systemic lupus erythematosus,
lead poisoning,	arsenical poisoning,
diphtheria,	leprosy.

15. Impairment of Vision

Impairment of vision may affect one or both eyes. It may be noticed by the patient or discovered by testing his eyes and examining his fields of vision. A *scotoma* is a blind patch in the field of vision.

Causes of impairment of vision

Corneal scarring
Cataract
Glaucoma
Injury to the eye
Detachment of the retina
Macular degeneration
Retinitis pigmentosa
Occlusion of retinal vessels
Papilloedema
Optic neuritis
Pituitary tumour
Trachoma
Onchocerciasis

Corneal scarring

The sight is impaired by scarring of the cornea following an ulcer in the central region of the cornea. The scar is visible as a white patch.

Cataract

A cataract is a degeneration of the normally transparent lens of the eye and is visible through the pupil as a white opacity. The whole lens is gradually involved, and there is a progressive impairment of eyesight going on to complete blindness. The degeneration can be the result of:

congenital diseases (e.g. maternal German measles),
metabolic disease (especially diabetes mellitus),
inflammation,
injury,
radiation by X-rays or infra-red rays.

Glaucoma

Impairment of vision can be due to glaucoma, a rise in the
intra-ocular pressure which produces degeneration of the
retina.

In *simple glaucoma* the pressure rises gradually over several
months, there is no pain, the eye appears normal, and the loss
of sight is so gradual that much can be lost before the patient
is aware of it.

In *acute glaucoma* there is a rapid rise in the pressure; the
patient has severe pain in and around the eye, is prostrated,
has nausea and may vomit. The cornea of the eye looks misty,
and oedema makes the iris look grey and patternless.

Injury

A blow to the eye may impair sight by:

(a) dislocating the lens out of its normal position,

(b) causing a cataract,

(c) interfering with retinal function and so causing a temporary loss of sight,

(d) causing a haemorrhage of the retina,

(e) tearing the retina and causing it to become detached.

Detachment of the retina

With this condition the patient notices a sudden loss of sight
in one eye. Detachment of the retina is usually due to either
(a) injury, or (b) high myopia, when the eyeball lengthens
and the sclera stretches more than the retina. The layer of
rods and cones becomes stripped off the choroid coat, from
which comes their blood supply, and the potential space
becomes occupied by vitreous humor. With complete detachment the eye becomes blind.

Macular degeneration

A degeneration of the macula of the retina, the area of highest visual sensitivity, causes a gradual impairment of sight. It occurs usually in old age. In *Tay-Sachs disease* (amaurotic family idiocy) it begins in infancy or childhood, goes on to cause complete blindness, and is associated with severe mental degeneration, paralysis and fits.

Retinitis pigmentosa

Loss of peripheral vision and night-blindness occur with retinitis pigmentosa, in which tiny star-shaped patches of black pigment appear in the retina, which degenerates. It starts in adolescence.

Occlusion of retinal blood vessels

Sudden blindness in one eye is produced by blocking of the central artery of the retina by spasm of its muscular wall, by atheromatous degeneration of its inner coat or by an embolus. Sight can return when the blindness is due to a spasm which passes off. Similarly, sudden blindness can be produced if the central vein of the retina is blocked by phlebitis or compressed by inflamed tissue around it; a slight recovery of sight—to the 'counting fingers' level—can occur if the acute condition settles down.

Papilloedema

A gradual blurring of vision is produced by papilloedema. Papilloedema is a swelling of the optic disc, and the commonest cause of it is a rise in intracranial pressure due to a tumour within the skull.

Optic neuritis

Impairment of sight is an early and severe symptom in this condition, with central vision being affected first. One or both eyes can be affected. Optic neuritis is an inflammatory condition of the optic nerve which goes on to degeneration of the myelin coat of the nerve fibres. Known causes are:

multiple (disseminated) sclerosis (recovery can occur
    when the inflammation settles down),
methyl alcohol,
tobacco smoking,
lead,
arsenical compounds.

The onset is usually acute. The patient complains of blurring
of vision, which gets worse for several days. Pain around the
eye is often complained of, may begin before the blurring of
vision, and is made worse by moving the eye. The patient
may have difficulty in judging distances.

Pituitary tumour

A bitemporal hemianopia can occur (i.e. visual impressions
coming from the side are not transmitted to the brain) if a
tumour of the pituitary gland grows forwards and presses on
the fibres which come from the nasal side of the retina and
cross in the optic chiasma.

Trachoma

This is a common cause of blindness in the Near East. It is a
chronic viral infection which produces blindness by causing
corneal scarring.

Onochocerciasis

This is a cause of blindness in certain parts of Africa, South
and Central America, and the Yemen. Blindness is due to
invasion of the eyes by the larvae of a filarial worm.

16. Impairment of Hearing

Impairment of hearing may be:

(a) *conductive*: sound waves are not conducted to the cochlea, i.e. the lesion is in the outer or middle ear;

(b) *perceptive*: a defect in the cochlea, auditory nerve or brain prevents auditory sensations from being appreciated.

Causes of impairment of hearing

Congenital disease
Wax, etc. in external auditory meatus
Otitis media
Injury
Virus infection
Otosclerosis
Ménière's disease
Acoustic neuroma
Senility
Noise
Drugs

Congenital disease

A child may be born deaf as a result of:

maternal German measles (rubella),
haemolytic disease of the newly born,
anoxia and birth injury,
some rare metabolic diseases affecting the brain.

Deafness may be associated with mental handicap, and it can be difficult to distinguish between a deaf baby and a mentally handicapped baby.

Wax, etc. in external auditory meatus

Deafness may be due to blocking of the external auditory

meatus by:

> wax,
> a boil, due to infection of hair follicles in the meatus,
> an exostosis, a bony outgrowth of the meatus,
> a foreign body.

Otitis media

(a) *Acute otitis media.* The patient is usually a child. He has a severe throbbing headache which can cause him to scream for hours. Deafness may be accompanied by tinnitus (a ringing noise in the ear). The patient will be flushed and have a raised temperature, and the eardrum will show evidence of acute inflammation and may become perforated.

(b) *Chronic otitis media.* This can follow an acute otitis media when it has not been treated in time or inadequately, when the patient is in poor general health, when the infection is a virulent one, or when there is chronic nasal or pharyngeal infection. Deafness is due to damage to the eardrum and middle ear. The perforation in the eardrum does not heal up and there is chronic discharge.

(c) *Secretory otitis media* (catarrhal otitis media, glue ear). Deafness, a 'stuffy feeling' in the ear, and sometimes slight transitory pain occur in this condition. There is an effusion of blood in the middle ear visible through the eardrum. It can be due to:

> repeated, inadequate antibiotic treatment of an acute
>   otitis media,
> adenoids,
> otitis barotrauma (see below).

Injury

Deafness can be due to:

(a) *rupture of the eardrum* due to a blow on the head, bomb blast, the noise of a jet engine, a firework or a fracture of the temporal bone.

(b) *otitis barotrauma,* usually due to landing rapidly in an unpressurized aircraft. The tympanic (Eustachian) tube collapses and does not allow air to enter the middle ear; the tympanic membrane is pushed inwards and cannot oscillate properly. A secretory otitis media can follow.

Virus infection

Sudden unilateral or bilateral deafness of the perceptive kind can follow an upper tract viral infection. The viruses most likely to cause it are those of:

> chickenpox,
> mumps,
> measles.

Patients in whom this kind of deafness has occurred have usually been adults.

Otosclerosis

Deafness is *the* feature of this disease in which new bone forms around the footplate of the stapes in the middle ear and by preventing it from vibrating interferes with the transmission of vibrations into the cochlea. Women are twice as often affected as men. The usual age of onset is 15–30 years and there is often a family history of deafness. It begins in one ear and then involves both. Paracusis (an ability to hear conversation more easily in noisy than in quiet surroundings) and tinnitus may be present.

Ménière's disease

Deafness occurs in Ménière's disease, in which there is a rise of pressure in the inner ear. The patient suffers attacks of giddiness, nausea and vomiting and has severe tinnitus (a ringing noise in the ear). The deafness is a perceptive one, is often worse just before and after an attack, is gradually progressive, and may be associated with gross distortion of normal sounds.

Acoustic neuroma

Deafness of gradual onset may be the first sign of an acoustic nerve tumour. This is a tumour of fibrous tissue growing in the sheath of the acoustic (eighth cranial) nerve and compressing it. The tumour may be a single one or part of a generalized neurofibromatosis (von Recklinhausen's disease). Deafness, tinnitus and giddiness are likely, and the fifth and seventh cranial nerves may be pressed on.

Senility

A perceptive deafness, due to cochlear dysfunction, is common in old age.

Noise

Deafness due to cochlear dysunction can be due to prolonged exposure to loud noise, as in certain industries or pop bands.

Drugs

Deafness due to damage to the auditory nerve is a side effect of some drugs, especially:

> streptomycin,
> salicylates,
> quinine.

17. Low Back and Leg Pain

Pain in the lower part of the back may stay there or radiate downwards into the legs. It can be due to:

certain general conditions,
lesions of the spinal column, cord and nerves.

1. GENERAL CONDITIONS

General conditions

Tiredness
Tension
Obesity
Menstruation
Pregnancy

Tiredness

Long periods of standing are likely to produce pain in the back, especially in a person who has some mild degree of spinal deformity—scoliosis, kyphosis or lordosis. Unsuitable postures, working practices or equipment can be causes of backache.

Tension

Backache is a common complaint of tense, anxious people.

Obesity

Obese people tend to get pain in the back because of the extra weight they carry, fatty infiltration of muscles, lack of muscle tone, lordosis, and stretching of the ligaments connecting the vertebrae.

Menstruation

Some women experience pain in the back during their menstrual periods.

Pregnancy

The different carrying-angle of the body and extra weight of baby, placenta, amniotic fluid and enlarged uterus can be a cause of backache in pregnancy.

2. LESIONS OF SPINAL COLUMN, CORD AND NERVES

Backache and pain in the legs are commonly due to structural changes in the spinal column, to collapse of diseased vertebrae, and to pressure on the spinal cord or nerves.

Lesions of spinal column, cord and nerves

Prolapse of lumbar intervertebral disc
Injury
Infection
Tumour
Ankylosing spondylitis
Spondylolisthesis
Osteoporosis of spine
Paget's disease of spine

Prolapse of lumbar intervertebral disc

In this condition the annulus fibrosus of an intervertebral disc ruptures at the back and the nucleus pulposus of the disc projects backwards through the opening and can press on the spinal nerves. It occurs in the cervical as well as in the lumbar region.

The patient is usually a young adult. When it occurs in the lumbar region it is usually the result of lifting a heavy weight.

The patient complains of a sudden pain in the back, a pain so intense that he may be unable to move. The pain shoots down the legs either immediately or some hours later, usually into the back of the thigh and the outside of the calf. The patient usually calls the pain in the back 'lumbago' and the pain in the legs 'sciatica'. The pain is made worse by coughing and sneezing and relieved by rest. In some patients pressure on the spinal nerves causes muscle weakness and paralysis, sensory loss and loss of the tendon reflexes.

Injury

Pain in the back can be due to injury to the spinal column, to a fracture or to stretching of the spinal ligaments. If lumbar nerves are pressed on, the pain radiates into the legs. Common fractures are:

> fracture of a transverse process,
> fracture-dislocation of the spine,
> crush-fracture of a vertebral body.

Infection

(a) *Tuberculosis of spine.* The patient is usually an adolescent or young adult. He complains of a gradually coming on and localized pain and of muscular spasm. A vertebral body is affected and can collapse. Complications are: (i) kyphosis due to collapse of the infected vertebral body; (ii) pressure on spinal cord and nerves; (iii) a psoas abscess, which is an abscess within the sheath of the psoas muscle;

(b) *Osteomyelitis.* Osteomyelitis can occur in a vertebra and cause pain in the back, pyrexia and malaise.

(c) *Typhoid fever.* A painful, stiff 'typhoid spine' can occur as a late complication of typhoid fever, and last for months. It is due to inflammation of the intervertebral discs, ligaments and periosteum.

Tumour

Pain and signs of pressure on the spinal cord or nerves may be due to a benign or malignant tumour. A malignant tumour is likely to be secondary to a primary growth elsewhere—usually in the breast, lung, prostate gland, kidney or thyroid gland. A sudden, severe pain in the back is felt if a pathological fracture occurs at the site of the tumour.

Ankylosing spondylitis

Morning stiffness and low backache are the first symptoms of this condition. It is a disease of unknown origin in which chronic inflammation and degeneration occur in the spine and sacro-iliac joints and sometimes in other joints. Affected joints become ankylosed, i.e. fixed together by bony outgrowths. The spine becomes increasingly rigid. The disease usually affects men in their thirties, but in can begin in childhood or adolescence and sometimes occurs in women. Iritis (inflammation of the iris of the eye) occurs in about 40 per cent of people affected.

Spondylolisthesis

A chronic low backache in a young adult can be due to this condition, which is thought to be the result of a congenital defect in which one vertebra (and all the spine above it) is moved forwards on the next one below it. It occurs most commonly in the lumbar region.

A similar slipping forward of one vertebra on the one next below it occurs in middle-aged or old people as a result of degenerative changes in the intervertebral disc, loss of disc substance, and narrowing of the disc space. The pain is relieved by movement or by sitting with a pillow in the small of the back, and is made worse by lifting or bending. It may spread into the leg, but more as a dull diffuse ache than a pain.

Osteoporosis of spine

A chronic low backache and stoop in an old person can be due to loss of calcium from a vertebra, the body of which becomes smaller and produces a kyphosis. An acute pain is produced when the vertebral body collapses.

Paget's disease of bone (osteitis deformans)

Low backache is a common symptom in this condition in which bone becomes first soft and enlarged and later hard and brittle. It occurs in middle or old age. Other features of it are enlargement of the head, kyphosis, bow legs and pathological fractures.

3. DISEASES OF ABDOMINAL ORGANS

Backache can be produced by some diseases of abdominal organs.

Diseases of abdominal organs

Pyelonephritis
Pancreatitis
Aneurysm of abdominal aorta
Gynaecological diseases

Pyelonephritis

Pain in the back can occur in pyelonephritis. The pain can be colicky or a dull ache in the loin. It is likely to be associated with frequency of micturition, pyrexia, rigors, malaise, vomiting, constipation and headache. The kidney is sometimes palpable and tender.

Pancreatitis

The pain of acute and chronic pancreatitis may radiate from the epigastrium to the back. In the acute state there is likely to be shock, vomiting and tenderness on deep palpation of the upper abdomen. The pain of chronic pancreatitis is at first less severe, but it can in time become more severe and almost continuous.

Aneurysm of abdominal aorta

Pain in the lower back radiating into the buttocks and legs can be produced by an atheromatous aneurysm of the abdominal aorta. A sudden exacerbation of pain may be a sign that the aneurysm is about to rupture. The aneurysm is sometimes palpable as a pulsating tumour in the abdomen.

In a *dissecting aneurysm of the aorta* a split occurs in the wall of the aorta, usually in the thoracic part of the aorta, and blood is forced into the wall and into the abdominal aorta. An agonizing pain in the chest spreads down the back as the aneurysm enlarges downwards. The patient is likely to be an old man. He suffers severe shock and may die on the spot.

Gynaecological diseases

A woman with pain in the back is more likely to be suffering from one of the conditions described above than from a gynaecological disease. Sometimes, however, the pain appears to be due to some condition within her pelvis.

(a) *Prolapse of uterus*. Backache in the sacral region sometimes occurs in this condition in association with a feeling of 'bearing down', frequency of micturition and stress incontinence.

(b) *Retroversion of uterus*. In this condition the uterus is bent backwards instead of forwards. Usually it causes no symptoms.

(c) *Chronic inflammation in the pelvis*. Backache sometimes occurs when the pelvic organs are chronically inflamed. The cause is usually gonorrhoea.

(d) *Large fibroid tumours and ovarian cysts*. A dull backache can occur or more severe pain radiating into the legs if the anterior branches of the sacral nerves are pressed on.

(e) *Malignant tumours*. Pain in the back and legs can be an indication that the anterior sacral nerves have been invaded by a malignant growth from a pelvic organ.

18. Loss of Appetite

Anorexia is an abnormal loss of appetite.

Causes of loss of appetite

Infection
Anxiety state
Anorexia nervosa
Depression
Malignant disease
Chronic alcoholism
Renal or hepatic failure
Simmonds' disease
Addison's disease
Drugs

Infection

Appetite can be lost in any infection, especially tuberculosis.

Anxiety state

Appetite is lost in an acute anxiety state. In chronic anxiety, however, the patient may overeat and become fat.

Anorexia nervosa

The appetite is lost in anorexia nervosa and the patient refuses to eat. It is an illness of young women, thought to be due to emotional stress and characterized by starvation, loss of weight, amenorrhoea and a downy growth of hair on the back. The patient remains active in spite of being thin and eating nothing. Pulmonary tuberculosis can develop.

Depression

A depressed patient is likely to lose his appetite or may

refuse to eat because he thinks he is unworthy to live, because he is deluded that he has no stomach or bowels, or because he decides on starvation as a method of committing suicide.

Malignant disease

Appetite is lost in any malignant disease. Characteristic of carcinoma of the stomach is a dislike of meat.

Chronic alcoholism

Appetite can be lost in chronic alcoholism as a result of the development of chronic gastritis, which produces nausea and vomiting, and of cirrhosis of the liver, early symptoms of which are nausea, vomiting and malaise.

Renal or hepatic failure

Loss of appetite occurs early in both renal and hepatic failure and can precede other clinical features.

Simmonds' disease (panhypopituitarism)

Loss of appetite is a feature of Simmonds' disease, in which there is a failure of pituitary function, usually as a result of an infarction of the gland after a severe obstetrical haemorrhage. Other features are weakness, apathy, amenorrhoea, atrophy of genitalia and loss of hair. There is a concurrent failure of thyroid and adrenal function owing to the lack of the pituitary hormones which are their normal stimuli.

Addison's disease

In this disease there is a failure of adrenal function usually due to an atrophy of the glands or their invasion by tuberculosis. The onset is usually insidious and the course slowly progressive. Loss of appetite is associated with malaise, loss of weight, tiredness, nausea, dehydration, and a light brown or brownish-black pigmentation of the skin.

Drugs

(a) *Digitalis*: loss of appetite is an early sign of overdosage by digitalis and should be particularly enquired for when a patient is undergoing digitalization.

(b) *Appetite-suppressant drugs*. Claims are made for various drugs that they suppress appetite and can be used in the treatment of obesity, but none of them appear to be very effective.

19. Difficulty in Swallowing

Causes of difficulty in swallowing

Local causes	sore throat
	foreign body in oesophagus
	carcinoma of oesophagus
	stenosis of oesophagus
	Plummer-Vinson syndrome
	achalasia
Pressure on oesophagus	malignant lymph nodes
	carcinoma of bronchus
	retrosternal goitre
	aneurysm of aorta
Other conditions	myasthenia gravis
	bulbar poliomyelitis
	diphtheria
	oesophageal spasm

LOCAL CAUSES

Sore throat

Difficulty in swallowing is experienced in tonsillitis and pharyngitis, after tonsillectomy, and after burning the throat with a corrosive liquid.

Foreign body in oesophagus

A pointed foreign body or a large rounded one can stick in the oesophagus and cause a painful difficulty in swallowing. The patient is likely to be a young child or a mental patient.

Carcinoma of oesophagus

The patient with a carcinoma of oesophagus develops a

progressive difficulty in swallowing—at first of solid food, then of semi-solid food, and finally of liquids. He is likely to be a middle-aged or old man and a heavy drinker. He can usually indicate on his chest the point at which food sticks. Pain in the chest or upper abdomen is common. Regurgitation of food, hoarseness and respiratory difficulty are less common.

Stenosis of the oesophagus

Difficulty in swallowing can be due to stenosis of the oesophagus. Stenosis is a fibrous contraction of part of the oesophagus following damage by a corrosive liquid, a foreign body, or a surgical operation.

Plummer-Vinson syndrome

Difficulty in swallowing is associated with an iron-deficiency anaemia. The difficulty in swallowing is due to a degeneration of the mucous membrane in the upper part of the oesophagus. The patient will be middle-aged or old and pale and may have a smooth tongue or spoon-shaped finger-nails.

Achalasia of the oesophagus

In this condition difficulty in swallowing and retrosternal discomfort are due to an inability to relax of the lower oesophageal sphincter (just above the stomach) and an absence of normal oesophageal peristalsis. Nerve cells in the oesophageal wall show signs of degeneration. It occurs in both sexes and at any age.

Pressure in the oesophagus

Difficulty in swallowing can be due to narrowing of the oesophagus by pressure from outside. The pressure can be due to:

> malignant lymph nodes, secondary to carcinoma of the breast, stomach, bronchus, etc.,
> carcinoma of the lung,
> retrosternal goitre, a goitre occuring in a thyroid gland abnormally situated behind the sternum,
> aneurysm of the thoracic aorta.

Other conditions

Difficulty in swallowing can be a symptom of *myasthenia gravis*, a condition in which muscles quickly become fatigued; of paralysis of the tongue and pharyngeal muscles in *diphtheria*, with regurgitation of food and fluid through the nose; and of paralysis of the pharyngeal muscles in *bulbar poliomyelitis*, when motor nerve cells in the medulla oblongata and pons of the brain are affected.

Oesophageal spasm causes a severe retrosternal pain, which lasts for about a minute and can be followed by soreness. Often it closely resembles pain produced by organic disease of the heart.

20. Abdominal Pain

Abdominal pain may be produced by diseases of the abdominal organs or by diseases of structures outside the abdomen.

The ways by which pain is produced from diseased abdominal organs are obscure.

Colic (colicky pain) is a painful spasm of any hollow muscular organ. It gets its name because it was originally applied to pain arising in the colon, but it is now applied to pain arising in other organs:

> intestinal colic: in the intestine, small and large
> appendicular colic: in the appendix
> biliary colic: in the biliary tract
> ureteric colic: in the ureter
> tubal colic: in the uterine (Fallopian) tube.

The pain is usually very severe and is often superimposed upon continuous pain. Attacks may be accompanied by vomiting. The patient may roll in agony or go into a state of shock.

Inflammation of the parietal peritoneum produces a severe, continuous pain localized over the inflammation and associated with local tenderness and muscular rigidity (guarding). Movement makes this pain worse.

Common sources of pain from abdominal organs

Stomach and duodenum:	acute gastritis
	peptic uler
	perforation of peptic ulcer
	carcinoma of stomach
Intestines:	intestinal obstruction
	appendicitis
	ulcerative colitis
	diverticulitis
	carcinoma of colon
	tuberculosis

Peritoneum:	peritonitis
	subphrenic abscess
Biliary tract:	acute cholecystitis
	chronic cholecystitis
	gall-stones
Pancreas:	acute pancreatitis
	chronic pancreatitis
Urinary tract:	acute pyelonephritis
	urinary calculus
	carcinoma of kidney
	acute cystitis
	urinary obstruction
Female genital system:	torsion of ovarian cyst
	haemorrhage into ovarian cyst
	torsion of fibroid tumour
	red degeneration of fibroid tumour
	acute salpingitis
	ectopic pregnancy
	abortion

1. STOMACH AND DUODENUM

Pain is caused by:

acute gastritis,
peptic ulcer,
perforation of an ulcer,
carcinoma of the stomach.

Acute gastritis

Acute gastritis is due to excessive consumption of aspirin, to swallowing a corrosive liquid or to infection. It produces epigastric pain, vomiting and loss of appetite.

Peptic ulcer

A peptic ulcer causes pain in the epigastrium and sometimes elsewhere. If the ulcer is in the stomach, the pain comes on 30–60 minutes after a meal; if it is in the duodenum, it comes on 3–4 hours after a meal and can wake a patient up from sleep. It is relieved by food, alkalis and vomiting. The mechanism by which the pain of peptic ulcer is produced is not definitely known; it has been attributed to the action of acid on the ulcer and to a muscular spasm in the stomach wall.

Perforation of a peptic ulcer

Perforation of a peptic ulcer into the peritoneal cavity produces a sudden and severe pain in the epigastrium; later the pain is felt over the whole abdominal wall. The patient goes into a state of shock, with collapse, a rapid feeble pulse, a grey complexion and sweating. The abdomen will have a board-like rigidity and the epigastrium will be acutely tender.

Carcinoma of the stomach

A carcinoma of the stomach is more likely to produce discomfort than pain, but pain can occur in the epigastrium and radiate into the back. The patient is likely to have lost weight and be anaemic, and the carcinoma may be felt as a hard mass in the upper abdomen.

2. INTESTINES

Intestinal obstruction

Intestinal obstruction is most commonly due to:

> strangulation of a hernia,
> intussusception,
> volvulus,
> Crohn's disease,
> chronic diverticulitis,
> carcinoma of the large intestine,
> impaction by faeces or a large gall-stone.

A colicky pain is usually the first symptom in any form of obstruction. When the obstruction is due to a strangulated hernia, there is a severe pain of sudden onset at the site of the hernia as well as a central colicky pain. The other symptoms of obstruction from any cause are: abdominal distension, absolute constipation (no faeces and flatus are passed), and vomiting. In some cases peristalsis is visible. When a strangulation is present, the temperature and pulse rate are raised.

Appendicitis

Typically the pain of acute appendicitis begins in the umbilical region and about six hours later moves to the site of the appendix—to the right iliac fossa when it lies there, to the suprapubic region when it hangs down into the pelvis, and to the right loin when it lies behind the caecum. The shift of the pain to the right iliac fossa is due to local involvement of the peritoneum. Movement makes the pain worse and the patient may find relief by lying with flexed knees. The onset of pain is quickly followed by nausea and vomiting. The abdomen is tender over the inflamed appendix and there is often some local rigidity (guarding) of the abdominal wall there. The patient is flushed and has a raised temperature and pulse rate. When the appendix hangs down into the pelvis, it may be tender to rectal examination.

Ulcerative colitis

Ulcerative colitis is an inflammation of the large intestine which occurs in a mild chronic form with long remissions, a severe chronic form or an acute fulminating form which can quickly be fatal. Cramp-like abdominal pain, varying in severity with the severity of the colitis, accompanies the attacks of diarrhoea with mucus, blood and pus in the stools.

Diverticulitis

Diverticulitis is inflammation of the diverticula which can occur in the colon, most commonly in the pelvic colon. The patient is usually an obese man over fifty. The diverticula do not cause pain until acute inflammation begins. Pain then occurs in the subumbilical region and moves into the left iliac fossa. The combination of left-sided pain with vomiting, local tenderness and muscular rigidity prompts the name of 'left-sided appendicitis'.

A dull or colicky pain occurs in the left iliac fossa in *chronic diverticulitis*, and the clinical condition then resembles that of carcinoma of the colon.

Carcinoma of the colon

The type of carcinoma of the colon likely to produce pain is the constricting variety in which the lumen of the intestine is progressively narrowed. This occurs usually in the left half of the colon. Colicky pain in the left iliac fossa can occur. Distension of the caecum can cause pain in the right iliac fossa. The patient is likely to be over the age of forty and to complain of irregularity of bowel action and of loss of weight and appetite. The carcinoma may be palpable through the abdominal wall or on rectal examination.·

Tuberculosis

Abdominal tuberculosis—of intestine and peritoneum—can cause colicky pain, vomiting, fever and menstrual disorders. Constipation is common. An abdominal mass may be palpable.

3. PERITONEUM

Peritonitis

The pain and other features of peritonitis is added to the symptoms and signs of the condition to which the peritonitis is due. This may be:

> perforating wound of the abdomen,
> traumatic rupture of bowel,
> perforation of a peptic ulcer,
> perforation of an acute appendix,
> acute cholecystitis,
> acute diverticulitis and perforation of a diverticulum,
> infection from an abdominal operation,

acute salpingitis,
puerperal infection,
septicaemia.

The onset of peritonitis is marked by a sudden, severe, generalized abdominal pain. The patient lies very still because any movement makes the pain worse. Other symptoms and signs are: vomiting, abdominal tenderness, slight distension, rigidity of the abdominal wall, absent abdominal sounds (listened for through a stethoscope), and a raised temperature and pulse rate. If the diaphragm is irritated by the peritonitis, the patient may experience pain in the shoulder due to the transmission of stimuli up sensory fibres in the phrenic nerve to the cervical cord.

Subphrenic abscess

A subphrenic abscess is an abscess in the space between the diaphragm and the liver. It is usually due to infection elsewhere in the abdomen. The usual symptoms are malaise, a swinging pyrexia, nausea, anaemia and loss of weight. The condition is not easy to diagnose unless some local symptoms are present as well. One of these is pain, which can occur in the upper abdomen or lower chest or be referred to the tip of the shoulder.

4. BILIARY TRACT

Pain arises in the gall-bladder and bile ducts from:

acute cholecystitis,
chronic cholecystitis,
gall-stones.

Acute cholecystitis

The pain of acute cholecystitis if felt below the right costal margin or in the epigastrium or as a band across the upper part of the abdomen; it can radiate to the back or to the right shoulder. It begins as a dull ache to which become added bouts of acute pain. Similar pain can be produced by perforation of a peptic ulcer, acute appendicitis, acute pancreatitis, and by coronary thrombosis and pneumonia of the base of the right lung, two chest diseases in which pain can be felt in the epigastrium. In acute cholecystitis the area is tender and the inflamed, distended gall-bladder can sometimes be felt as a rounded tender mass projecting below the right costal margin.

Chronic cholecystitis

The pain of chronic cholecystitis is an intermittent pain in the same area as the pain of acute cholecystitis. A feeling of fullness in the same area is common.

Gall-stones

Biliary colic is the pain produced by the impaction of a gall-stone in the outlet of the gall-bladder or in the common bile duct and is agonizing. It can radiate from the right subcostal region and epigastrium to the lower angle of the right scapula. It stops if the stone falls back into the gall-bladder or is forced through the sphincter of Oddi into the duodenum. A stone impacted in the common bile duct obstructs the flow of bile into the duodenum and causes an obstructive jaundice within a day or two. As stones are likely to be associated with chronic cholecystitis, some dull pain is likely to be present between attacks of biliary colic.

5. PANCREAS

Pain can arise in the pancreas as a result of:

      acute pancreatitis,
      chronic pancreatitis.

Acute pancreatitis

The pain of acute pancreatitis is a severe pain in the epigastrium or upper left quarter of the abdomen; it can radiate to the back. It can last for several days. It is likely to be associated with vomiting, shock and tenderness on deep palpation of the upper part of the abdomen. In this condition patches of pancreatic tissue are destroyed apparently by pancreatic enzymes in the pancreatic juice, and the pain is due to the haemorrhages and oedema which develop in the gland.

Chronic pancreatitis

The pain of chronic pancreatitis is at first less severe than that of acute pancreatitis, but as the disease progresses more and more areas of gland are destroyed and the pain becomes severe and almost continuous.

6. URINARY TRACT

Pain can arise in the urinary tract as a result of:

> acute pyelonephritis,
> urinary calculus,
> carcinoma of the kidney,
> acute cystitis,
> urinary obstruction.

Acute pyelonephritis

The pain of acute pyelonephritis is a dull pain in one of both loins, and is associated with frequency of micturition, fever, tenderness in the loin, and cloudy and sometimes blood-stained urine.

Urinary calculus

A very severe pain with sharp exacerbations occurs when a renal stone becomes impacted at the junction of the pelvis ureter or is squeezed by muscular contractions down the ureter. The pain is called ureteric colic. It radiates from the back to the groin, to the left iliac fossa or to the external genitalia. It can last for hours, with the patient in a state of shock or rolling in agony. A large stone embedded in the kidney substance does not cause pain, and a small stone in the pelvis of the kidney which is not being forced into the ureteric opening may cause only a dull pain in the loin.

A stone in the bladder produces pain in the suprapubic region or the perineum. At the end of micturition the pain is sometimes felt in the end of the urethra.

Carcinoma of the kidney

A dull pain in the loin can be produced by a carcinoma of the kidney. Urinary colic can occur if blood from the tumour clots and blocks the ureter.

Acute cystitis

Pain in the suprapubic area is produced by an acute cystitis and is associated with frequency of micturition. There may be pain in the loin if the patient also has an associated pyelonephritis.

Urinary obstruction

Urinary obstruction occurs in men. It can be due to:

> enlargement of the prostrate gland,
> carcinoma of the prostrate gland,
> urethral stricture,
> impaction of a stone in the opening of the bladder into the urethra.

A severe pain in the suprapubic region is produced by an acute retention with a sudden enlargement of the bladder, but there is little or no pain if the obstruction is a gradual one.

7. FEMALE GENITAL SYSTEM

Pain can arise in the female genital system as a result of:

> torsion of ovarian cyst,
> haemorrhage into ovarian cyst,
> torsion of fibroid tumour,
> red degeneration of fibroid tumour,
> acute salpingitis,

ectopic pregnancy,
abortion.

Torsion of ovarian cyst

A sudden severe abdominal pain is caused if the stalk of an
ovarian cyst becomes suddenly twisted and the blood vessels
in it are compressed, the cyst itself becoming swollen with
blood. The patient may go into a state of shock and will have
a tender and rigid abdomen. A milder pain is produced by a
gradual torsion. Torsion is particularly liable to occur when
the abdominal wall is relaxed, as after pregnancy.

Haemorrhage into ovarian cyst

Any haemorrhage into an ovarian cyst, with distension of its
wall, will cause abdominal pain, severe if the haemorrhage is
sudden, mild if it is gradual.

Torsion of fibroid tumour

Acute abdominal pain is caused if a fibroid tumour of the
uterus attached to it by a stalk undergoes torsion (twisting),
in which there is a sudden interference with its blood supply.
The patient may vomit and go into shock.

Red degeneration of fibroid tumour

Abdominal pain, vomiting and fever occur if a fibroid tumour
of the uterus undergoes a form of degeneration called red
degeneration in which it becomes a pinkish-red and swollen
due to thrombosis occurring in its blood vessels. It occurs
most commonly during pregnancy.

Acute salpingitis

Lower abdominal pain can be due to an acute infection of
the uterine tube (gonorrhoea is the commonest cause) and is
associated with irregular menstrual bleeding, malaise and fever.
The lower abdomen is tender and there is some muscular
rigidity (guarding) there. Sometimes it occurs only on one

side and when the side is the right side, the diagnosis from acute appendicitis is difficult and sometimes impossible.

Ectopic pregnancy

Lower abdominal pain occurs when a pregnancy develops in the uterine tube. It is at first slight and irregular, later more severe and constant and becomes most severe when the tube ruptures. The patient collapses from shock and haemorrhage.

Abortion

Pain is not a feature of 'threatening abortion' when bleeding is the symptom, but if the 'threatened abortion' proceeds into an 'inevitable abortion' rhythmical, lower abdominal pains occur due to the contractions of the uterus.

SOURCES OF PAIN FROM OUTSIDE THE ABDOMEN

Sources of pain from outside the abdomen

Angina pectoris
Coronary thrombosis
Diaphragmatic pleurisy
Herpes zoster
Spinal tumour
Spinal root compression
Tabes dorsalis
Lead poisoning
Psychiatric causes

Angina pectoris and coronary thrombosis

The pain of angina pectoris and of coronary thrombosis may be referred to the epigastrium. The milder pain of angina pectoris is often attributed by the patient to indigestion. The severe pain of coronary thrombosis when it is felt in the epigastrium may be thought to be due to an acute abdominal emergency.

Diaphragmatic pleurisy

Pain can occur in the epigastrium or upper abdomen from a pleurisy at the base of a lung, where the pleura lies immediately above the diaphragm.

Herpes zoster

Herpes zoster, a viral infection involving the sensory ganglion of a spinal nerve, causes irritation and pain in the distribution of the nerve to the skin. If the nerve involved belongs to segments Thoracic 8–12, the pain or irritation is felt in a band which runs from the back to the midline in front and slightly downwards. The pain may precede the development of the typical rash in the same band. Pain may persist for weeks, months or years in the affected part.

Tumour of the spinal cord

A tumour of the spinal cord occurring in the lower thoracic region of the cord can produce pain in a girdle round the trunk. The pain is intermittent and made worse by moving, jolting, coughing and straining.

Spinal root compression

Abdominal pain can be caused by spinal root compression. The pain is segmental and tenderness or altered sensation can occur in the same area. The pain is sometimes increased by tensing the abdominal muscles or moving the spine.

Tabes dorsalis

Tabes dorsalis, a late syphilitic disease of the spinal cord, can produce: (a) burning or constricting pain around the trunk (b) visceral crises, in which acute abdominal pain is associated with vomiting; crises of this kind are rare, but when one occurs it can be mistaken for an acute abdominal emergency.

Lead poisoning

Lead poisoning can produce intestinal colic, usually in the umbilical region. The condition may be 'mistaken for an acute abdominal emergency. The patient is likely to complain of weakness, fatigue, constipation and muscular pains. The poisoning can be due to the absorption of lead in an industrial process, to children licking lead-containing paint, or to a workman bringing home lead on his clothes, person or car.

Psychiatric causes

Recurrent or persistent abdominal pain occurs in depression, chronic tension and chronic alcoholism. In school children recurrent abdominal pain is often emotionally determined.

21. Vomiting

Causes of vomiting

Abdominal diseases
Infections
Diseases of the nervous system
Diseases of the ear
Mental states
Kidney disease
Diabetic crisis
Gynaecological conditions
Allergy
Drugs
Poisons

ABDOMINAL DISEASE

Vomiting is a common feature of many acute and chronic abdominal diseases.

Abdominal diseases

Acute and chronic gastritis
Peptic ulcer
Carcinoma of the stomach
Pyloric stenosis
Intestinal obstruction
Acute appendicitis
Acute peritonitis
Acute cholecystitis and gall-stones
Renal calculus
Acute pancreatitis

Acute and chronic gastritis

Vomiting is an early feature of acute gastritis, an acute irritation of the mucous membrane of the stomach commonly due to alcohol or food poisoning. It is associated with nausea, lack of appetite, and abdominal discomfort, and a little later with diarrhoea if there is also an enteritis.

Peptic ulcer

Vomiting can occur with a gastric or duodenal ulcer and tends to relieve the pain of the ulcer. It is likely to be present when there is a stenosis of the pylorus following the healing (with the formation of scar tissue) of an ulcer in the pyloric region.

Carcinoma of the stomach

Vomiting can be a feature of carcinoma of the stomach when the growth is in the pyloric region and blocks the escape of food into the duodenum.

Pyloric stenosis

Projectile vomiting (in which the vomit shoots out of the mouth) in the second or third week of life is the presenting feature of congenital hypertrophy of the pylorus, and can occur with pyloric stenosis or blocking in later life.

Intestinal obstruction

Vomiting occurs in intestinal obstruction from any cause (see p. 89).

Vomiting occurs early if the obstruction is in the small intestine, and later or not at all if it is in the large intestine. The vomit is at first colourless; later it becomes brown and foul-smelling due to altered blood and the decomposition of the contents by bacteria. (True faecal vomiting, i.e. the vomiting of faeces, occurs only when there is a fistula between the stomach and the colon, a cancer of the stomach growing into the colon or a cancer of the colon growing into the stomach.)

Acute appendicitis

Nausea and vomiting are usually present in acute appendicitis and begin after the onset of pain in the umbilical region. The vomiting is not usually severe except in young children.

Acute peritonitis

Frequent vomiting is likely to occur in acute peritonitis from any cause. It will be associated with severe pain, localized or generalized tenderness, and abdominal rigidity. With a prolongation of the peritonitis, the vomiting can become faeculent.

Acute cholecystitis and gall-stones

Nausea and vomiting are common features of acute cholecystitis and of biliary colic due to impaction of a gall-stone in a hepatic or biliary duct.

Renal calculus

Vomiting can occur with renal colic due to the impaction of a renal calculus in the ureter.

Acute pancreatitis

Vomiting is a feature of acute pancreatitis and is associated with severe upper abdominal pain, epigastric tenderness, and sometimes shock.

INFECTIONS

Nausea and vomiting commonly occur in some infections and usually early. They are likely in the following infections:

acute poliomyelitis   Vomiting is common and is likely to be associated with fever and pain in back and limbs and in some cases with paralysis.

bacillary dysentery	Vomiting can accompany the diarrhoea.
benign myalgic encephalo-myelitis (Royal Free Hospital disease)	Vomiting occurs in about half the cases and is associated with lassitude, malaise, sore throat, etc.
cholera	Sudden, explosive vomiting of clear infectious fluid can occur.
epidemic vomiting	An acute viral infection of which vomiting is the main feature; it lasts for 2–3 days and several members of a family can be affected at the same time.
food poisoning	Vomiting is associated with diarrhoea and abdominal pain in all types of food poisoning.
meningitis and encephalitis	Associated with fever, headache and stiffness of the neck.
scarlet fever	Vomiting is associated with headache, fever, a sore throat and a rash.
smallpox	Vomiting is common and associated with fever, rigors, headache, pain in the back and a rash.
whooping cough	Vomiting is brought on by bouts of coughing.

DISEASES OF THE NERVOUS SYSTEM

Vomiting can be due to increase in intracranial pressure. In *cerebral haemorrhage* vomiting can occur before the onset of coma. With a *cerebral tumour* vomiting is associated with headache, early attacks being sometimes called 'bilious attacks' by the patient; it is usually due to the increase in intracranial pressure produced by the tumour, but sometimes it is due to the local effects of a tumour of the cerebellum or to a tumour pressing on the eighth cranial nerve.

DISEASES OF THE EAR

Motion sickness

Vomiting is the essential feature of any motion sickness (car sickness, sea sickness, plane sickness).

Ménière's disease

In this condition nausea and an uncontrollable vomiting commonly occur during the paroxysmal attacks of giddiness and tinnitus (ringing in the ears).

MENTAL STATES

Vomiting can occur in:
> fright and anxiety,
> anorexia nervosa,
> hysteria.

Fright and anxiety

Some people vomit at the sight of blood, injured people, etc., or in a stress-provoking situation.

Anorexia nervosa

The patient is usually a young woman who develops a profound loss of appetite, starves herself and becomes emaciated. If forced to eat, she may vomit.

Hysteria

Vomiting can be one of the ways in which a person with hysteria can react.

DISEASES OF THE KIDNEY

Acute nephritis type 1 (acute haemorrhagic nephritis)
Nausea, vomiting, diarrhoea and abdominal pain can precede

renal symptoms such as pain in the back, oedema, reduced renal output and haematuria, or occur at the same time.

Renal failure

Nausea and vomiting are among the gastro-intestinal symptoms of renal failure and are likely to persist.

DIABETIC CRISIS

Vomiting can be a feature of diabetic crisis (diabetic coma) and can make it worse by increasing the loss of fluid and electrolytes.

GYNAECOLOGICAL CONDITIONS

Vomiting can be due to:

> dysmenorrhoea,
> acute salpingitis,
> torsion or red degeneration of a fibroid tumour of the uterus,
> torsion of an ovarian cyst,
> rupture of an ectopic pregnancy

Hyperemesis gravidarum is a severe vomiting which occurs during pregnancy and has been attributed to hormonal changes (it can occur before the patient knows she is pregnant) or possibly to a psychological rejection of the pregnancy. It usually clears up on admission to hospital and correction of fluid and electrolyte imbalances.

ALLERGY TO FOOD

Some patients are allergic to certain foods and react to them by vomiting, having diarrhoea, or developing urticaria. They usually know what they are sensitive to, but they may unwittingly take some of it in a dish of whose contents they are ignorant.

DRUGS

Drugs can produce vomiting (a) by irritating the mucous membrane of the stomach, (b) in a person who is hypersensitive to a particular drug, or (c) as an indication of overdosage. Among the many drugs which can for one reason or another produce vomiting are:

aminophylline	tetracylines
acetylsalicylic acid	ammonium chloride
(aspirin)	colchicine
codeine phosphate	PAS
digitoxin	pethidine
levodopa	phenylbutazone
morphine	sulphonamides
potassium iodide	oral contraceptives
stilboestrol	

POISONS

Vomiting can be due to:

excessive consumption of alcohol,
acute arsenical poisoning,
poisoning by iron compounds,
poisoning by toadstools,
exposure to radioactive substances.

HAEMATEMESIS

Haematemesis is the vomiting of blood. The patient usually knows he has vomited. The amount of blood may be slight or large and it may be mixed with gastric juice or food. 'Coffee grounds' is the name given to small amounts of brown partly digested blood.

Haematemesis is due to bleeding from:

multiple small peptic ulcers due to aspirin
peptic ulcer
carcinoma of stomach
oesophageal varices (dilated veins at the junction of
    oesophageal and stomach liable to occur in cirrhosis
    of the liver)
surgical operations on the throat, etc., when some
    blood has been swallowed.

22. Diarrhoea

Diarrhoea may be acute or chronic; acute exacerbations of a chronic diarrhoea can occur. In some conditions (carcinoma of colon, irritable colon) constipation may alternate with diarrhoea.

Causes of diarrhoea

Bacterial infection	bacillary dysentery
	staphylococcal food poisoning
	typhoid, paratyphoid fever
	cholera
Parasites	amoebic dysentery
	roundworms
	tapeworms
	hookworms
	Giardia lamblia
Diet	rhubarb, plums
	alcohol
Malabsorption	steatorrhoea
	coeliac disease
	sprue
	Crohn's disease
	bowel resection and short circuits
Drugs	purgatives
	digitalis
	antibiotics
Neoplasm	carcinoma of colon
Poisons	arsenic
Kidney disease	chronic renal failure
Other conditions	anxiety
	irritable colon syndrome

ulcerative colitis
thyrotoxicosis

Bacterial infection

The diarrhoea of *bacillary dysentery* can be slight or severe according to the degree of severity of the infection, and is associated with vomiting, generalized colicky abdominal pain, and fever. The diarrhoea of *staphylococcal food poisoning* comes on suddenly, is severe, can cause shock and dehydration, and lasts usually for only a few hours. The diarrhoea of *typhoid fever* begins during the second week of the disease, after a period of constipation, and continues for the rest of the attack; the stools are fluid and pale yellow. The diarrhoea of *paratyphoid fever* is less severe than that of typhoid fever. The diarrhoea of *cholera* is sudden and extremely severe, with the patient passing numerous 'rice water' stools and becoming dehydrated.

Parasites

Amoebic dysentery occurs in inhabitants of tropical countries, immigrants from them and travellers to them; it can occur in an acute and a chronic form. In the acute form the diarrhoea is severe and associated with colicky lower abdominal pain, slight fever, and blood and mucus in the stools; in the chronic form diarrhoea is associated with flatulence and some colic and with mucus in the stools. Mild diarrhoea can sometimes be produced by *roundworm* and *tapeworm* infestation. Diarrhoea, anaemia and cachexia develop in *hookworm* infestation. *Giardia lamblia* infection is a common cause of diarrhoea.

Diet

Some people develop diarrhoea after eating rhubarb or plums. Loose stools or diarrhoea can be due to an excessive consumption of alcohol.

Malabsorption

Chronic diarrhoea and malnutrition occur as results of a failure of absorption of essential food factors by the small intestine. Such malabsorption occurs in:

> coeliac disease,
> idiopathic steatorrhoea,
> tropical sprue,
> Crohn's disease (regional ileitis),
> resection or short circuit of the small intestine.

Drugs

Drugs which cause diarrhoea are:

> any purgative,
> digitalis: diarrhoea—along with nausea, vomiting, slow pulse, doubling of beats—is a sign of overdose,
> antibiotics: antibiotics can cause diarrhoea by interfering with the normal bacterial content of the bowel.

Neoplasms

Diarrhoea, constipation or alternating diarrhoea and constipation occurs with *carcinoma of the colon*. With a constriction growth, more common on the left side, signs of intestinal obstruction are likely; and with a cauliflower growth, more common on the right side, blood is likely to be present in the stools.

Poisons

Severe diarrhoea and vomiting occur in *acute arsenical poisoning*.

Other conditions

Mild diarrhoea is commonly due to *anxiety*. An irregular bowel action—with spells of diarrhoea, constipation, flatulence, colicky pain, and the passage of mucus—occurs in the *irritable colon sydrome.* Diarrhoea is the principal symptom of *ulcerative colitis*; it is present in all phases of the illness, varying in severity with the degree of severity of the disease, which can be acute, chronic or mild; the stools contain blood and mucus; and during the remissions of the disease some looseness of the bowels is likely. Some diarrhoea can occur in *hyperthyroidism*, in association with an enlarged thyroid gland, exophthalmos, tremor, sweating and palpitations.

23. Constipation

Constipation may be due to a single factor or to a number of factors acting together, such as senility and lack of food.

Causes of constipation

Habit and diet	lack of bulk in food starvation dehydration dyschezia
Hypothyroidism	myxoedema cretinism
Mental states	depression senility mental retardation
Organic diseases	carcinoma of colon diverticulitis fistula-in-ano haemorrhoids
Drugs	opium, morphine, belladonna, atropine

Habit and diet

Constipation can occur when the faeces are too small to excite defaecation. This happens in *starvation*, in *dehydration* when the faeces are small because of lack of fluid, and as a result of a *lack of bulk* when the food does not contain adequate amounts of bran (present in wholemeal bread) and fibres (present in green vegetables). *Dyschezia* is constipation due to a persistent refusal to answer the call to empty the bowels.

Hypothyroidism

Constipation is a feature of the two hypothyroidic conditions, *cretinism* and *myxoedema*, in which there is an inadequate secretion of thyroid hormone and all metabolic process are diminished

Mental states

Constipation is a feature of *severe depression*, as a result of reduced peristalsis, indifference to the call to empty the bowels, and depressive ideas that the bowels do not exist or cannot be opened. Constipation is common in *senility* as a result of a combination of factors: reduced appreciation of the need to empty the bowels, indifference, reduced food intake, lack of bulk in the diet, physical weakness, and difficulty in getting to a lavatory. Constipation is common in *mental retardation* when the mentally retarded person cannot be trained to empty the bowels.

Organic disease

Constipation can alternate the diarrhoea in a case of *carcinoma of the colon* and *diverticulitis*. It is liable to occur when defaecation is painful and avoided as with *fistula-in-ano* and *thrombosing haemorrhoids*.

Drugs

Constipation can be caused by drugs which reduce peristalsis:

opium	morphine
belladonna	atropine

24. Blood in the Stools

Blood can appear in the stools as:

(a) *melaena*: this is blood which has been acted upon by the digestive juices and become black and 'tarry'. (Like some other words in medicine, e.g. melanin, melanotic, melaena is derived from the Greek word *melas – melanos*: black).

(b) *bright red blood*: this comes either from the lower part of the alimentary tract or as a massive haemorrhage from the upper part which stimulates peristalsis and is passed before the digestive juices can act upon it.

Causes of blood in the stools

Swallowed blood
Oesophageal varices
Peptic ulcer
Acute gastric erosions
Carcinoma of stomach
Jejunal polyp
Typhoid fever
Mesenteric artery thrombosis
Ulcerative colitis
Carcinoma of colon or rectum
Haemorrhoids

Swallowed blood

Blood may be swallowed during a dental or nasal operation or from an injury to the mouth.

Oesophageal varices

Oesophageal varices can bleed and cause haematemesis and blood in the stools. They are dilated veins at the oesophageal-gastric junction, the dilation being due to cirrhosis of the liver.

Peptic ulcer

A gastric or duodenal ulcer can bleed and cause haematemesis or blood in the stools. The bleeding is usually slight and appears as melaena, but a massive haemorrhage can occur if a large blood vessel becomes eroded by the ulcer.

Acute gastric erosions

Bleeding can occur from an acute gastric erosion, which can be due to stress, taking aspirin, acute infection or a severe burn. The bleeding is slight and appears as melaena.

Carcinoma of stomach

Slight bleeding takes place from the surface of a carcinoma of the stomach and causes melaena. The patient is likely to be anaemic and will be losing weight; the liver may be enlarged from secondary growths in it, and a hard malignant lymph node is sometimes palpable just above the left clavicle, which carcinomatous cells have reached via the thoracic duct.

Jejunal polyp

This is an uncommon benign growth of the jejunum which can produce a massive haemorrhage.

Typhoid fever

Bleeding can occur during the second or third week of typhoid fever from ulcerated Peyer's patches in the small intestine, and can be followed by perforation through the bowel wall into the peritoneal cavity. Bleeding is slight and causes melaena.

Mesenteric artery thrombosis

Bleeding into the bowel can follow the clotting of blood in one of the arteries supplying the intestine.

Ulcerative colitis

Bleeding commonly occurs from the ulcers of the colon in this condition, which is characterized by attacks of diarrhoea with blood and mucus in the stools. The severity of the disease can vary from a mild condition with slight bleeding to a severe toxic state with much bleeding, fever, anaemia and prostration. Remissions are followed by relapses.

Carcinoma of colon or rectum

Ulcerated carcinomas of the colon or rectum produce bright red blood in the stools or alone.

Haemorrhoids

Bleeding is a common feature of haemorrhoids.

25. Jaundice

Jaundice is a yellow colour of the skin, sclerotics of the eyes and mucous membranes, and is due to an excessive amount of bilirubin in the plasma of the blood. The normal amount of bilirubin in the plasma is less than 15μmol/1 (1mg per 100ml). Jaundice comes detectable when the amount rises above 35μmol/1 (2mg per 100ml).

Bilirubin is a pigment which passes into the blood when red blood cells are destroyed. Red blood cells live for about 120 days and are broken down in the liver, spleen and bone-marrow. Bilirubin circulates in the blood until it arrives in the liver. It is taken out of the blood by the liver cells and converted by them into another form which is then excreted in the bile. When the bilirubin arrives in the small intestine, it is there converted into stercobilinogen. Stercobilinogen is the pigment which gives to the stools their typical colour.

Types of jaundice

1. Haemolytic jaundice: due to excessive destruction of red blood cells
2. Hepatic jaundice: due to malfunction of the liver
3. Obstructed jaundice: due to obstruction in the biliary tract.

---

1. HAEMOLYTIC JAUNDICE

Haemolytic jaundice occurs in:

      acholuric jaundice,
      sickle cell anaemia,
      malaria and some other infections,
      when an incompatible blood transfusion has been given.

The jaundice is slight because there is only a slight increase in the amount of bilirubin in the blood. The colour of the stools is normal.

2. HEPATIC JAUNDICE

This jaundice is partly due to inability of the cells of the liver to take bilirubin out of the plasma and convert it into the form in which it is excreted in bile, partly to stagnation of bile in the canaliculi (the small channels in the liver along which the bile passes to get to the larger biliary ducts), and some reabsorption of the bilirubin. It occurs:

> in some infections, especially infective hepatitis, yellow fever, leptospirosis, infective mononucleosis, septicaemia,
> as a toxic effect of certain drugs: chlorpromazine, chloroform, cincophen, gold, thioracil, etc.

The stools are pale.

3. OBSTRUCTIVE JAUNDICE

Obstructive jaundice is caused by:

> impaction of a gall-stone in the common bile duct,
> carcinoma of the head of the pancreas,
> carcinoma of the ampulla of Vater,
> chronic pancreatitis.

The dammed-up bile is reabsorbed via the lymph vessels into the blood. The jaundice becomes progressively deeper and may turn green. The stools are pale because no stercobilinogen is formed and have an offensive smell because the absence of bile interferes with the digestion of fat.

26. Epistaxis

Epistaxis (nose bleeding) can be due to local or general conditions. The bleeding is usually from a small area at the front of the septum. It can be slight or serious and even fatal.

LOCAL CAUSES

Local causes

'Spontaneous' epistaxis
Trauma
Foreign body
Tumour
Atrophic rhinitis
Hereditary telangiectasis

'Spontaneous' epistaxis

This is an epistaxis likely to occur and recur in children and young people and easy to stop. It is sometimes due to infection or slight injury, but sometimes there is no obvious cause.

Trauma

Epistaxis may be due to a punch on the nose or a surgical operation on it.

Foreign body

Epistaxis may be due to a pointed foreign body or to attempts to remove one. The patient is likely to be a child, a mentally retarded person or a mental patient.

Tumour

Epistaxis or a blood-stained discharge can be due to a malignant tumour of the nose or wall of the maxillary sinus.

Atrophic rhinitis

Epistaxis, an unpleasant smell and headache can be due to atrophic rhinitis, a degeneration of the mucous membrane of the nose.

Hereditary telangiectasis

Epistaxis can be due to bleeding from a naevus in the nose in this condition, in which naevi develop there, on the lips and tongue, and in the alimentary tract.

GENERAL CONDITIONS

General conditions

Infections
Hypertension
Haemorrhagic diseases
Drugs

Infections

Epistaxis can occur at the beginning of any severe infection, especially:

> influenza,
> meningococcal septicaemia,
> smallpox,
> typhoid fever.

Hypertension

A severe epistaxis can occur in hypertension of any kind, and if severe may temporarily improve the condition of the patient.

Haemorrhagic diseases

Epistaxis can occur in any disease of which bleeding is a feature, especially:

purpura,
leukaemia,
haemophilia,
scurvy,
vitamin K deficiency.

Drugs

Epistaxis can occur as a side effect of:

quinine,
salicylates,
Sedormid.

27. Palpitations and Shortness of Breath

PALPITATION

Palpitation is awareness of the heart's action. Normally one is not aware of one's heartbeats except after exertion, but one can become aware of them in certain conditions, especially:

    extra systoles,
    atrial fibrillation,
    paroxysmal tachycardia,
    atrial flutter.

(a) *Extra systoles.* An extra systole is a premature contraction (ectopic beat) of the heart resulting from an impulse which has arisen from some site in the heart other than the normal one (the sinu-atrial node). After an extra systole there is a long pause before the next beat occurs due to the suppression of the next normal beat. The patient may not notice an extra systole, but he may be aware of having missed a beat or complain of thumping in the chest or of what he calls his heart 'turning over'.

(b) *Atrial fibrillation.* In this condition the ventricles of the heart contract rapidly and irregularly, some patients being aware of the rapidity and irregularity. The pulse is irregular in both rhythm and volume. Signs of heart failure may be present.

(c) *Paroxysmal tachycardia* (atrial tachycardia). In this condition paroxysms of rapid beating of the heart occur. The rate is usually 150–220 times a minute. Paroxysms begin and end suddenly, last from minutes to days, and recur in irregular intervals. The patient complains of severe palpitations, which come on without warning, of pain in the precordial region, and of faintness and giddiness.

(d) *Atrial flutter.* This condition is less common than the above. In it the atria beat at about 180–360 times a minute, but the ventricles cannot keep up this speed and beat at about 160–180 times a minute. The patient has usually got an organic disease of the heart. He complains of palpitations, precordial pain, faintness and giddiness.

SHORTNESS OF BREATH

Shortness of breath occurs when the oxygen content of arterial blood falls below that needed for the functioning of the tissues.

Dyspnoea is a noticeable increased effort in breathing. It can vary from a physiological dyspnoea produced temporarily on exertion to a dyspnoea that is present at rest and prevents the patient from making any effort. *Orthopnoea* is a dyspnoea made worse by lying down and relieved by sitting up or standing.

Causes of shortness of breath

Disease of the heart
Disease of the lung
Disease of the blood
Other conditions

Disease of the heart

Shortness of breath occurs in heart failure—when the heart fails to pump out enough blood to provide the tissues with the oxygen they need. Common causes of heart failure are:

valvular disease of the heart,
myocardial infarction (due to coronary thrombosis),
atrial fibrillation,
paroxysmal tachycardia,
pericarditis (a pericardial effusion or a constrictive pericarditis interferes with cardiac function and prevents the return of venous blood to the heart),
chronic disease of the lungs.

Disease of the lung

Shortness of breath occurs when diseases of the lung interfere with the oxygenation of blood or with normal respiratory movements. It is to be expected in:

> pneumonia,
> asthma,
> spontaneous pneumothorax,
> bronchitis, acute and chronic,
> emphysema,
> collapse of lung,
> fibrosis of lung.

(a) *Pneumonia.* In pneumonia from any cause the patient will be acutely ill, with rapid respiration and a raised pulse rate and temperature.

(b) *Asthma.* The patient will have painful, wheezy respirations due to spasm of the bronchial muscle.

(c) *Spontaneous pneumothorax.* In this condition a pleural cavity suddenly fills with air due to the rupture into it of a cyst in the lung. Sudden dyspnoea and chest pain occur. The patient is usually a previously healthy young man, and the presence of a cyst in his lung has been unsuspected.

(d) *Bronchitis.* In acute bronchitis dyspnoea is due to swelling of the mucous membrane of the bronchi and the presence of excessive secretion in them. In chronic bronchitis, which is often associated with emphysema, the patient is likely to have wheezing breath sounds, shortness of breath and dyspnoea.

(e) *Emphysema.* In this condition distension of the alveoli interferes with normal respiration. Dyspnoea is the outstanding symptom. Cyanosis of the lips and cheeks is often present, and the chest becomes barrel-shaped and hyper-resonant.

(f) *Collapse of lung.* Shortness of breath comes on suddenly if a bronchus is blocked by a foreign body, by mucus or by a clot of blood, and slowly when obstruction is due to carcinoma of a bronchus or to pressure on it by malignant lymph nodes.

(g) *Fibrosis of lung.* Shortness of breath is due to interference with the passage of gases through the walls of the alveoli.

Disease of the blood

Shortness of breath occurs when an anaemia is so severe that insufficient oxygen is carried to the tissues because of shortage of red blood cells or of an inadequate concentration of haemoglobin in them. It can occur in:

> severe blood loss,
> iron-deficiency anaemia,
> pernicious anaemia,
> haemolytic anaemia,
> aplastic anaemia,
> leukaemia.

Other conditions

Shortness of breath can be due to:

(a) *exertion*: this is normal and should cease at the end of the exertion.

(b) *anxiety*: some people respond to stress by rapid breathing.

(c) *hysteria*: panting and over-breathing can be manifestations of hysteria.

(d) *pregnancy, ascites or distension of the abdomen from other causes*: pressure on the diaphragm can produce shortness of breath.

28. Pain in the Chest

Pain in the chest can arise in various structures.

Sources of pain in the chest

Muscles of the chest wall
Ribs
Heart
Pericardium
Pleura
Oesophagus and stomach
Spinal column
Nerves
Hyperventilation

Muscles of the chest wall

Two kinds of pain arise in the muscles of the chest wall: a dull continuous pain or severe stabbing pain lasting a few seconds. Some patients complain of both. The pain is felt all over the chest or in the lower left chest. Attacks may occur daily for weeks or months and then cease, sometimes to recur later. No definite cause is known; they are usually called rheumatic or fibrotic pains. Occasionally muscular pain is due to tearing a muscle in strenuous exercise.

Ribs

Fracture of a rib or ribs is due to a direct blow, to compression of the chest or rarely to a violent fit of coughing. Pain over the site of the fracture is produced by coughing, sneezing or deep breathing or by movements of the trunk or arm on the same side.

Heart

Pain arising in the heart may be:

angina pectoris
due to coronary thrombosis

Angina pectoris is a pain which comes on usually when the patient is engaged in some physical activity—climbing stairs, climbing a hill, walking quickly or against a wind, carrying a heavy bag, etc. Occasionally it occurs at rest. Emotional stress can bring it on and smoking makes it worse. It is due to a shortage of blood supplied to the myocardium when the coronary arteries are partly blocked by atheroma or constricted by spasm in the muscle of the wall of the artery. The pain begins usually in the precordial region, the part of the chest in front of the heart. It may stay there or radiate to the left side of the chest, occasionally to the right side, down the left arm, into the neck and jaw, into the back, or into the epigastrium, the upper central part of the abdominal wall. It usually stops the patient from carrying on with his activity, although some patients try to 'walk through' it. It clears up spontaneously or can be stopped, as well as prevented, by taking glyceryl trinitrate, a drug which dilates the coronary arteries. In some patients the attacks of pain occur at rest and without emotional crises; in them attacks tend to recur in a regular pattern and be prolonged.

Coronary thrombosis, a clotting of blood in an atheromatous coronary artery, causes a pain similar to that of angina pectoris, but much more severe. The patient may have had attacks of angina pectoris. Shock, nausea and vomiting are likely, and about one patient in four dies either immediately or within ten days.

Pericardium

A dull continuous pain over the lower end of the sternum can be due to:

> infections (viral, tubercular) of the pericardium,
> invasion of the pericardium by carcinoma of lung.

The patient is likely to discover that the pain is relieved if he sits up and leans forward. A pericardial rub, caused by the rubbing together of the two layers of the pericardium, can be heard through a stethoscope. The patient may also have a pleurisy.

Spontaneous pneumothorax

A spontaneous pneumothorax produces pain in the chest and dyspnoea (see p. 124).

Pleurisy

Pleurisy causes a sharp pain in the side or centre of the chest. It is made worse by deep breathing, coughing and sneezing, and the patient may hold his side to prevent it from moving. The pain is relieved if a pleural fluid develops and separates the two layers of pleura. The pleurisy can be due to:

> pneumonia,
> cancer of the lung invading the pleura,
> embolism of the pulmonary artery.

Pleural friction causes a typical sound which can be heard with a stethoscope and is due to the rubbing together of the two inflamed surfaces.

Oesophagus and stomach

Pain in the front of the chest can be due to:

> carcinoma of the oesophagus,
> hernia of the stomach through the diaphragm,
> peptic ulcer.

In *carcinoma of the oesophagus* a dull pain is felt in the front of the chest and is associated with difficulty in swallowing. A *hernia of the stomach* (hiatal hernia) through a defect in the diaphragm produces a dull pain in the chest, least when he is standing and the stomach has fallen into the abdominal cavity, worst when he is laying down and it rises up into the thoracic cavity; the pain is relieved by vomiting. The pain of a *peptic ulcer* is sometimes felt in the chest or back instead of the abdomen; it tends to come on 30–60 minutes after a meal when it is in the stomach and 2–3 hours after a meal when it is in the duodenum, and is relieved by vomiting.

Spinal column

A dull continuous pain, made worse by movement of the head and liable to radiate down the arms into the hands, can be due to arthritic changes in the cervical vertebrae. There may be some limitation of movement in the neck, and bony outgrowths are visible on an X-ray.

Nerves

Herpes zoster, a viral infection involving the sensory ganglion of a spinal nerve, causes irritation of pain in the distribution of the appropriate nerve. Symptoms are felt in the segment supplied by the nerve, in a band running round and slightly down the chest from front to back. The condition is usually on one side, but can be on both. The patient is likely to be over the age of fifty. The pain can precede the development of the typical rash in the segment. Pain in the affected part may persist for weeks, months or years after the attack.

In *tabes dorsalis* (locomotor ataxia), a late syphilitic infection of the nervous system, girdle pains, encircling the body, can be felt.

Hyperventilation

The pain produced by hyperventilation can closely resemble the pain of organic heart disease. Some people are habitual hyperventilators, many of them practising breathing exercises in order to improve their athletic or singing performances. The pain is of mixed type (sharp, stabbing, aching, shooting, etc.) with a widespread and inconstant distribution (precordial and submammary areas, axillae, upper chest, shoulders, radiating to the arms and neck). It can last from seconds to days. It is likely to be associated with anxiety, palpitations, paraesthesiae in the arms and elsewhere. It is relieved or stopped by a return to a normal breathing pattern.

29. Fainting

Syncope is the medical name for a faint—a sudden and brief loss of consciousness following a sudden temporary reduction in the blood supply to the brain. It can be mistaken for a minor epileptic fit. If it is prolonged, a major fit can occur.

The syncope is due to certain circulatory changes. At the time of fainting the pulse is slowed, the blood vessels of muscles and internal organs are dilated and blood accumulates in them, and the BP falls so low that not enough blood reaches the brain. The skin is pale because the blood vessels in it are constricted.

Types of syncope

Reflex syncope
Postural syncope
Anoxic syncope
Micturition syncope
Cough syncope
Stokes-Adam syndrome
Syncope due to other heart diseases
Carotid sinus syncope
Areflexic syncope
Psychogenic fainting

Reflex syncope (vasovagal attacks)

This type of syncope is particularly noticeable in blood donors towards the end of the operation, after a period in which attempts to keep the BP high are made by increasing the pulse rate and constricting all blood vessels.

Postural syncope

Fainting occurs in some people when they stand up quickly. It is most commonly experienced by young adults, and more commonly by men than women. It tends to stop in time on its own accord, but some people with it have later developed temporal lobe epilepsy.

Anoxic syncope

Syncope due to a low oxygen content of the blood can occur when flying in an unpressurized aircraft and during the administration of nitrous oxygen for dental operations on patients sitting up.

Micturition syncope

This occurs in men who get up at night to pass water and is due to a sudden change in posture plus straining to initiate micturition. It is prevented by sitting for a few moments on the edge of the bed before standing up.

Cough syncope

This is syncope occurring during a bout of coughing. The patient usually has emphysema or chronic bronchitis. It is due to interference with the return of venous blood to the heart by a sudden raising of the intra-thoracic pressure.

Stokes-Adam syndrome

This is syncope due to heart block, the cardiac impulse failing to reach the ventricles from the atria. The pulse is slowed to 10–20 times a minute as the ventricle beats at its own inherent rate. Loss of consciousness can last up to a minute, and in prolonged attacks the patient develops sterterous or Cheyne-Stokes breathing and can have a fit.

Syncope due to other heart diseases

Syncope can occur in:

      congenital heart disease,
      rheumatic heart disease,
      aortic stenosis,
      any cardiac arrhythmia.

Carotid sinus syncope

This is a syncope produced by slight pressure on the neck over the bifurcation of the common carotid artery. It occurs in old people and may be due to some atheroma at the site.

Areflexic syncope

This is a syncope due to an interference with the reflexes which control the rate of the heart and the resistance of blood vessels and so control the supply of blood to the brain. It occurs in:

> tabes dorsalis,
> diabetic neuropathy and other kinds of neuropathy,
> patients taking phenothiazine drugs.

Psychogenic fainting

Pain, fear, the sight of blood, photographs of a bad accident, etc. can cause some people to faint. Psychogenic fainting is used by neurotic or unstable people to draw attention to themselves or to manipulate a situation. Multiple fainting can occur in groups of people as a result of standing for a long time, being exposed to sunshine, and seeing others faint.

30. Nasal Catarrh

Nasal catarrh is an excessive discharge from the mucous membrane of the nose.

Causes of nasal catarrh

Common cold (acute coryza)
Hay fever (seasonal allergic rhinitis)
Non-seasonal allergic rhinitis
Vasomotor rhinitis
Rhinitis due to drugs
Occupational rhinitis
Nasal polyps

Common cold (acute coryza)

This is a common cause of nasal catarrh and is due to an acute virus infection of the nasal mucous membrane.

Hay fever (seasonal allergic rhinitis)

The patient develops a blocked and running nose, sneezing and itchy red eyes as a result of sensitisation of the nasal mucous membrane to an allergen. In Britain the condition occurs in April–July, the common pollens being those of trees (April–May) and grass (June–July). Skin testing may identify the allergen.

Non-seasonal allergic rhinitis

This rhinitis is usually an allergic reaction to the house-dust mite, human hair or fabrics. When it is due to the dust mite it is usually worse when the patient is in bed, bedclothes being a place favoured by the mite.

Vasomotor rhinitis

This is a nasal catarrh of uncertain origin. It is said to be a manifestation of stress, especially in young people.

Rhinitis due to drugs

Drugs which can cause nasal catarrh in some people include:

> female sex hormones
> reserpine (Serpasil)
> nasal decongestants (as a 'rebound' effect)

Occupational rhinitis

Nasal catarrh can be produced in farmers by moulds and dusts, in welders by hot metal fumes, and in others who work with human hair.

Nasal polyps

Nasal polyps cause rhinitis and nasal obstruction and sometimes sinusitis.

31. Sore Throat

Sore throat is usually due to an infection of the pharynx and tonsils, and is an early feature of some common communicable diseases.

Causes of sore throat

Tonsillitis
Quinsy
Common cold
Scarlet fever
Diphtheria
ECHO virus infection
Influenza
German measles (rubella)
Mumps
Vincent's angina
Secondary syphilis
Infective mononucleosis
Agranulocytosis

Tonsillitis

In *acute tonsillitis*, a streptococcal infection, sore throat is likely to be associated with difficulty in swallowing, headache, general malaise, and sometimes earache. The tonsils are swollen and red; the tongue is furred; cervical lymph nodes are enlarged and tender. The patient, who is usually a child, has a raised temperature and flushed cheeks.

In *chronic tonsillitis* the patient is likely to complain of recurring sore throats and a constant urge to clear the throat.

Quinsy (peritonsillar abscess)

This is an abscess lying behind the upper pole of the tonsil and pushing the tonsil downwards and medially. It occurs as a complication of acute tonsillitis. The patient is ill, has a raised temperature, and complains of sore throat, difficulty in swallowing and earache.

Common cold

Sore throat can sometimes be a symptom of a common cold.

Scarlet fever

Sore throat, headache, vomiting and a raised temperature are early features of scarlet fever, which is a streptococcal infection of the throat with a rash. The tonsils and adjacent issues are reddened and a white or yellow mucopurulent exudate appears on the tonsils and can form a continuous membrane. The rash, an erythema with red spots, occurs within 24–48 hours of the onset.

Diphtheria

Some soreness of the throat occurs when diphtheria involves the fauces, but it is not a predominant feature and some children do not complain of it. Other features in the early stages are malaise, tiredness, headache, and a moderately raised temperature. A membrane, formed of secretions, fibrin and white blood cells, forms on the tonsils and adjacent tissues, and cannot be removed without leaving a bleeding area.

ECHO virus infection

Sore throat can be a feature of any ECHO virus infection. Other features which can occur are nausea, vomiting, diarrhoea, rashes of various kinds, and evidence of meningitis or encephalitis.

Influenza

Sore throat and a cough can follow the sudden onset of headache, shivering, pain in the limbs and a raised temperature which occur at the onset of influenza.

German measles (rubella)

A sore throat, headache, conjunctivitis, and a slight rise of temperature may be the first symptoms of German measles, and are followed by a blotchy rash and enlarged cervical or other lymph nodes.

Mumps

A slight sore throat can occur early in mumps and precede the swelling of the parotid glands, which is the typical feature of the infection.

Vincent's angina

Sore throat, painful swallowing and an offensive breath occur in Vincent's angina, an acute infection of the throat thought to be due to two micro-organisms, a spirochete and a spindle-shaped organism.

Secondary syphilis

A sore throat—uncomfortable rather than painful—can occur in the secondary stage of syphilis. Irregular, meandering ulcers called 'snail-track ulcers' occur on the fauces. Other features of secondary syphilis likely to be present are: a rash, enlarged lymph nodes, and a slightly raised temperature.

Infective mononucleosis (glandular fever)

Sore throat can occur with fever, malaise, headache, enlarged lymph nodes, jaundice in a few cases, and sometimes various rashes.

Agranulocytosis

Sore throat is a feature of this condition in which by the action of certain drugs on the blood-forming tissues there is a sharp fall in the number of granulocytes in the blood and in consequence a lowering of the body's resistance to infection. Reddening and ulceration of the throat, lips and mouth occurs, with fever, malaise, prostration and sometimes jaundice. Drugs which can produce the condition include:

anticonvulsants,   thiouracil,
antihistamines,   tranquillisers,
carbimazole,   sulphonamides.

32. Hoarseness

Hoarseness is due to disease of the larynx or of the nerves supplying the laryngeal muscles.

Causes of hoarseness

Laryngitis
Tuberculosis of larynx
Secondary syphilis
Benign tumour of larynx
Carcinoma of larynx
Keratosis laryngitis
Myxoedema
Damage to recurrent laryngeal nerve

Laryngitis

A painful hoarse croak or complete loss of voice occurs in *acute laryngitis*. There may be other signs of upper respiratory tract infection, and the larynx is sometimes painful and tender.

Hoarseness, cough, voice fatigue and a constant urge to clear the throat occur in *chronic laryngitis*.

Tuberculosis of larynx

Hoarseness or loss of voice can be due to tuberculosis of the larynx, secondary to tuberculosis of the lung. Patches of tuberculous tissue and ulceration follow infection of the laryngeal mucous membrane. The condition is seen in people whose pulmonary tuberculosis has not been diagnosed or has been inadequately treated.

Secondary syphilis

Hoarseness can be due to oedema of the vocal cords when the larynx is involved in secondary syphilis. Other signs of secondary syphilis likely to be present are: a rash, sore throat, enlarged lymph nodes, slight temperature.

Benign tumour of the larynx

Hoarseness can be due to a benign tumour of the larynx, but this is a rare tumour.

Carcinoma of larynx

A persistent hoarseness is the first and characteristic symptom of carcinoma of the larynx. Other features likely to occur are cough, slight haemoptysis, and with spread of the tumour pain on swallowing, difficulty in breathing, and earache (by referred pain). This is the most serious condition to affect the larynx. The patient is likely to be over 50 years old and a man; and any man of the right age who develops a persistent hoarseness should be seen by an ENT surgeon.

Keratosis laryngitis (leukoplakia of larynx)

A persistent hoarseness is produced by this uncommon condition in which patches of white tissue appear on the vocal cords.

Myxoedema

A hoarse croaking voice can be heard in myxoedema due to a myxoedematous thickening of the vocal cords. The patient will show other features of myxoedema: obesity, coarsening of the features, loss of hair, oedema of the legs, mental dullness and a dry skin.

Damage to recurrent laryngeal nerve

The right and left recurrent laryngeal nerves (which are branches of the vagus nerves) supply most of the muscles of the larynx. Damage to them produces hoarseness. This damage can be due to invasion by a carcinoma of the lung or as a hazard of thyroidectomy. An aneurysm of the aorta can damage the left recurrent laryngeal nerve, which loops round it.

33. Cough

Cough is a reflex intended to clear the respiratory tract of any obstruction. It is produced by irritation of the respiratory passages by gases, infections, excessive secretion, etc. Sensory impulses are conveyed to a centre in the medulla oblongata of the brain, whence motor impulses are sent to the muscles of respiration whose sudden contraction produces a cough.

Causes of cough

Irritation of the mucous membrane of the respiratory tract
Some communicative diseases
Diseases of the nasal and respiratory passages
Pressure on the respiratory passages
Diseases of the lung
Diseases of the heart
Psychogenic cause

Irritation of the mucous membrane of the respiratory tract

Cough can be due to:

smoking,
atmospheric pollution,
inhalation of irritant gases and fumes.

Prolonged exposure to these will cause chronic pharyngitis and laryngitis and a chronic dry cough. The cough may be associated with hoarseness.

Communicative diseases

(a) *Whooping cough.* Bouts of coughing and cold-like symptoms herald an attack of whooping cough. The bouts of coughing become more severe and then end in a whoop. The cough and whoop may persist for several weeks after other symptoms have cleared up.

(b) *Measles.* Cough, fever, sneezing, watery eyes and general misery are early symptoms. The rash does not appear until the fourth day.

(c) *Influenza.* A dry cough is common in influenza, usually beginning a day or two after the onset, which is characterized by fever, malaise, aches and pains, and shivering.

Diseases of the nasal and respiratory passages

Cough is a common symptom of diseases of the nasal and respiratory passages. With diseases of the nose and nasal sinuses it is set up by secretions of pus trickling down the back the throat. It can occur in:

adenoids,
chronic sinusitis,
virus infections of the throat,
pharyngitis,
laryngitis,
tuberculosis of the larynx,
carcinoma of the larynx,
chronic bronchitis,
foreign body in trachea or bronchus.

Pressure on the respiratory passages

Pressure on the trachea and bronchi from outside them can cause a cough. The pressure can be due to:

an enlarged thyroid gland,
malignant growths in lymph nodes,
aneurysm of the thoracic aorta.

Diseases of the lung

Cough is a feature of many diseases of the lung, especially:

tuberculosis,	carcinoma of lung,
bronchiectasis,	emphysema,
asthma,	pneumonia,
pneumoconiosis,	sarcoidosis,

farmer's lung and similar diseases.

Diseases of the heart

Diseases of the heart can cause a cough if they produce congestion of the lungs and excessive secretion in the intrapulmonary respiratory passages. Cough is likely to occur especially in:

> mitral stenosis,
> left ventricular failure.

Psychogenic cause

Some people have a dry little cough which becomes worse at times of stress.

Haemoptysis

Haemoptysis is the coughing up of blood. The amount may be small or large, depending on the size of the blood vessel from which it comes. The patient knows he has coughed it up. The blood is bright red and may be frothy.

Causes of haemoptysis

Rupture of blood vessel during coughing from any cause
Acute and chronic bronchitis
Carcinoma of lung
Pulmonary tuberculosis
Bronchiectasis
Abscess of lung
Mitral stenosis
Pneumonia
Infarction of lung

Haemorrhage from inflamed mucosa causes blood-stained purulent sputum in acute respiratory infections and in infective exacerbations of chronic bronchitis. Fungal infection of a healed tuberculous cavity is a fairly common cause of haemoptysis.

34. Haematuria

Haematuria is blood in the urine.

The amount of blood may be:

(a) microscopic: the urine appears normal and blood cells are detected on microscopic examination

(b) slight: the urine has a smoky appearance

(c) macroscopic: the blood gives the urine a bloody appearance.

The blood can come from any part of the urinary tract.

Causes of haematuria

Injury
Calculus
Diseases of the kidney
Diseases of the bladder
Diseases of the prostate gland
Diseases of the urethra
Haemorrhagic diseases
Some drugs

Injury

Haematuria can be due to:

(a) a tear of the kidney into the renal pelvis,

(b) rupture of the bladder by a fracture of the bony pelvis,

(c) rupture of the urethra.

Calculus

Haematuria can be produced by a calculus in the pelvis of the kidney, in the ureter and in the bladder. If the calculus is embedded in the substance of the kidney, the patient may not

144

have any symptoms. Haematuria is likely if the stone is impacted in the pelvi-ureteric junction or attempting to move down the ureter, and it will then be associated with ureteric colic. If the stone is in the bladder, haematuria will be associated with frequency of micturition and pain in the suprapubic region, the perineum or the tip of the penis; haematuria tends to occur at the end of micturition as the bladder contracts down upon the calculus.

Diseases of the kidney

(a) *Nephritis type 1* (acute glomerulonephritis). The urine is smoky or bloody; occasionally the blood has darkened or forms a reddish-brown precipitate. Urinary output is reduced. The patient is usually young and has had an acute streptococcal throat infection 1–3 weeks previously. He is likely to complain of fever in the loins, malaise and headache, has a slight fever, and develops oedema of the face, legs and external genitalia.

(b) *Nephritis type 2* (chronic parenchymatous nephritis). Microscopic blood may be present in the urine. The chief features of this type of nephritis are oedema and albuminuria.

(c) *Tuberculosis of the kidney.* Haematuria can be the first symptom of tuberculosis of the kidney. It is usually slight, and in many cases it does not occur. Frequency of micturition is the usual symptom.

(d) *Tumours of the kidney.* Haematuria can be due to:
  i. nephroblastoma; a malignant tumour of the kidney occurring most commonly during the first two years of life
  ii. carcinoma of the kidney: occurs in adult life.

A painless haematuria is most likely to be due to tumour of the kidney (or elsewhere in the urinary tract). There may be no other symptoms, but with the development of the malignant disease, the patient will develop abdominal pain and an abdominal mass.

(e) *Infarction of the kidney.* Microscopic haematuria can occur in bacterial endocarditis as a result of small infarcts produced by emboli from diseased heart valves, and its identification is a useful diagnostic point.

Diseases of the bladder

Haematuria can be due to a tumour of the bladder of which the commonest are:

    papilloma,
    carcinoma.

A painless haematuria is often the first symptom. A carcinoma can produce painful micturition and frequency and urgency of micturition.

Schistosomiasis (an infection of the bladder by a blood fluke) is a cause of haematuria in Egypt, other parts of Africa and some parts of South America.

Diseases of the prostate gland

(a) *Simple hypertrophy of the prostate gland.* Haematuria can occur usually at the end of micturition from congested veins in the mucous membrane of the bladder. The patient is a man over 50. The usual complaints are of frequency of micturition, difficulty of micturition and a feeble stream; retention of urine can occur.

(b) *Cancer of the prostate gland.* Haematuria can occur as in simple hypertrophy. In addition to the symptoms of obstruction the patient is likely to be in poor health and to be losing weight. On rectal examination the gland is found to be much harder than normal. Secondary deposits may be present in bone.

Diseases of the urethra

Haematuria can be due to a caruncle (a fleshy growth in the urethra of women) or to a naevus.

Haemorrhagic diseases

Haematuria can be a symptom of any disease in which bleeding is a feature, especially:

    haemophilia,
    purpura,
    leukaemia.

Drugs

Haematuria can be caused by some drugs, especially the anticoagulants such as heparin, phenindione, warfarin.

35. Enlargement of Lymph Nodes

Normal lymph nodes are soft and cannot be felt through the skin. In certain diseases they become swollen, harder and palpable.

Enlargement of lymph nodes is local or general. When local it is usually due to local sepsis or malignant disease, but it can be the beginning of some general disease. Other tissues in the body in which lymph tissue is present (e.g. the spleen) are often enlarged at the same time as the lymph nodes.

The principal sites in which diseased lymph nodes are felt are:

anterior triangle of neck,
posterior triangle of neck,
axilla,
inguinal region.

Lymph nodes within the chest may show as a shadow on an X-ray. Lymph nodes within the abdomen may become palpable if a number of them become matted together to form a large mass.

Enlarged lymph nodes may be:

(a) discrete: they can be felt individually.

(b) matted: they become attached to one another by disease processes.

Causes of enlarged lymph nodes

Infection
Malignant disease
Sarcoidosis
Chronic lymphocytic leukaemia
Hodgkin's disease
Connective tissue disease

INFECTION

Enlargement of lymph nodes occurs in several infections.

Acute streptococcal infection of pharynx, tonsils, ear

Enlarged cervical lymph nodes become palpable in the anterior triangle of the neck. In recurrent tonsillitis the nodes often remain enlarged between attacks.

Staphylococcal infection

Lymphangitis (inflammation of lymph vessels) and enlarged nodes can be caused by staphylococcal infection of the skin and subcutaneous tissue. Lesions of the fingers are likely to cause enlargement of the axillary lymph nodes. The glands can mat together and an abscess can form in the mass and discharge through the skin.

Tuberculosis

Enlarged lymph nodes can occur in the cervical, thoracic and abdominal regions and indicate a spread of tuberculous infection from a primary site in the throat, lungs or intestine. Typical tuberculous inflammation occurs in the nodes; caseation can occur and a 'cold abscess' can form and discharge through the skin. There are no signs of acute inflammation and the enlarged nodes are painless.

Syphilis

Local enlargement of lymph nodes draining the chancre occurs in *primary syphilis*; as the chancre is usually on the genitalia, the inguinal nodes on one or both sides are the nodes most commonly affected. There are no signs of acute inflammation: the nodes are neither tender nor painful, and the skin over them is not reddened. General enlargement of nodes, especially those in the posterior triangle of the neck, occurs in *secondary syphilis*; the nodes are discrete, india-rubber-hard and not tender.

Infective mononucleosis (glandular fever)

A local or generalized enlargement of lymph nodes occurs, in association with fever, headache, malaise, and an enlarged spleen. Abnormal mononuclear cells are found in the blood.

German measles (rubella)

Discrete, slightly enlarged and slightly tender lymph nodes are a feature of this infection. They are usually to be found in the posterior triangle of the neck.

Benign myalgic encephalomyelitis (Royal Free Hospital disease)

Slight enlargement of cervical lymph nodes in the posterior triangle of the neck is a feature of this infection, in association with fever, upper respiratory tract infection, neckache, backache, and emotional disturbance.

Cat-scratch fever

Local lymph nodes draining the scratch can become enlarged and painful and can suppurate in this infection produced by the stratch of a cat. The local enlargement is followed by a general enlargement of nodes in many parts of the body.

Cytomegalovirus infection

Enlarged lymph nodes can occur in one of the adult forms of this virus infection, in association with fever and hepatitis.

Toxoplasmosis

Enlarged lymph nodes are a feature of the 'lymphatic' form of toxoplasmosis, which usually occurs in children of 5–15 years.

Plague

A 'bubo'—a mass of painful, inflamed matted nodes—is the characteristic feature of bubonic plague.

MALIGNANT DISEASE

Carcinoma

One of the favoured ways by which carcinoma can spread is along lymph vessels into the lymph nodes draining the organ in which the carcinoma forms. Their appearance is therefore a sign that the carcinoma has spread from its original site. Affected lymph nodes feel hard.

Site of nodes	*Source of carcinoma*
cervical nodes	carcinoma of tongue, lip, pharynx, breast (by extension from the axilla); a small malignant node just above the left clavicle can occur in carcinoma of the stomach by spread up the thoracic duct
axillary nodes	carcinoma of breast
abdominal nodes	carcimoma of stomach, large intestine, body of uterus
sacral nodes	carcinoma of cervix of uterus

Lymphosarcoma

A sarcomatous growth can appear in many lymph nodes but most commonly in the cervical, mediastinal and abdominal nodes. Usually there is an obvious enlargement of a goup of nodes. It occurs in middle age and more commonly in men than women.

Sarcoidosis

Enlargement of lymph nodes, usually in the neck, can occur in this disease of unknown origin in which tubercles develop but do not caseate like those of tuberculosis. The nodes are discrete and not tender. Spontaneous remission can occur.

Chronic lymphocytic leukaemia

In this form of leukaemia enlarged lymph nodes, which may be local or general, are associated with weakness, malaise and anaemia. There is a greatly increased number of lymphocytes in the blood.

Hodgkin's disease (lymphadenoma)

The appearance of a number of enlarged lymph nodes is usually the first sign of this disease. The usual site is the neck; less commonly the axillary, thoracic and abdominal nodes are affected first, rarely the inguinal nodes. A characteristic feature is that the nodes become painful only when the patient takes any alcohol. Fever, malaise, anaemia, loss of weight, enlargement of the liver and spleen occur, and in time many organs and tissues are involved in the disease process.

Connective tissue disease

Enlargement of lymph nodes can be a feature of:

> systemic lupus erythematosus,
> rheumatic arthritis of children,
> Felty's syndrome.

(a) *Systemic lupus erythematosus.* Lymph nodes become enlarged at one time or another in about half the patients affected with this condition. The enlargement is sometimes due to a secondary infection.

(b) *Rheumatic arthritis of children* (Still's disease). Enlargement of lymph nodes can occur in this condition (which occurs in children under 16 years of age) in association with polyarthritis, malaise, a rash, pericarditis, etc.

(c) *Felty's syndrome.* In this condition enlargement of lymph nodes and of the liver and spleen occurs as a complication of severe rheumatoid arthritis.

36. Disorders of Menstruation

Menstruation normally begins between 10 and 17 years. Ninety-five per cent of girls have begun to menstruate before the age of 16. If a girl has not menstruated by the age of 18, it is unlikely that she will ever menstruate spontaneously. Menstruation is preceded 1–2 years earlier by a spurt of growth, the development of breasts and the growth of pubic hair.

AMENORRHOEA

Amenorrhoea can be:

> primary or
> secondary.

PRIMARY AMENORRHOEA

Primary amenorrhoea is said to have occurred when a girl has not menstruated by the age of 18. It is classified into:

(a) primary amenorrhoea with no secondary sex characteristics (breasts, pubic hair, libido),

(b) primary amenorrhoea when secondary sex characteristics have been present for two years.

Primary amenorrhoea with no secondary sex characteristics

Delayed puberty
Turner's syndrome
Congenital disturbance of hypothalamus-pituitary complex
Destruction of ovaries
Premature menopause

Delayed puberty

Rarely puberty occurs after 18 years.

Turner's syndrome

In this condition the patient is short; has a webbed neck (a fold of skin running down each side of the neck from head to shoulder), a broad chest and a wide carrying-angle of the arms; and may have a congenital disease of the heart. On chronosome examination she is found to have only one X chromosome instead of the normal two. As a result of this deficiency the ovaries fail to develop.

Congenital disturbance of the hypothalamus - pituitary complex

Amenorrhoea can be due to an absence of hormone production by the hypothalmus-pituitary complex. Various clinical types are described:

(a) *Lorain type*: the patient does not grow to adult size nor develop secondary sex characteristics.

(b) *Laurence-Moon-Biedl syndrome*: amenorrhoea is associated with blindness (due to retinitis pigmentosa), obesity, mental retardation, and absence of secondary sexual characteristics.

(c) *Fröhlich's syndrome* (dystrophia adiposogenitalis): the child remains short and becomes obese; the genitalia do not develop.

Destruction of ovaries

The ovaries can be damaged and destroyed by:

> mumps,
> tuberculosis,
> X-rays.

Premature menopause

In this condition the ovarian follicles (for some unknown reason) degenerate before the girl reaches puberty.

Primary amenorrhoea with secondary sex characteristics
Congenital abnormalities of genital tract
Testicular feminization
Masculinizing syndromes

Congenital abnormalities of the genital tract

Amenorrhoea can be due to:

(a) *hypoplasia of the uterus*: the uterus remains at an infantile state of development.

(b) *Stenosis of the uterus, complete transverse septum of the vagina, imperforate hymen*: in any of these conditions, menstruation occurs but the menstrual fluid cannot escape as the way out is blocked.

Testicular feminization

In this condition of hormonal imbalance, the person has the physical appearance of a woman but has little pubic and axillary hair. The gonads are testes, which are present within the abdomen or in the inguinal canal, and the sex chromosomes are the XY of the normal male.

Masculinizing syndromes

In these conditions there is a preponderance of male sex hormones. They can occur before or after puberty.

(a) *Polycystic ovaries* (Stein-Leventhal syndrome): the patient is obese and hairy and her kidneys are cystic and unusually large.

(b) *Adrenal hyperplasia*: there is an overproduction of androgens by an enlarged adrenal cortex.

SECONDARY AMENORRHOEA

Secondary amenorrhoea is amenorrhoea occurring after menstruation has begun.

Secondary amenorrhoea

Pregnancy
Menopause
Contraceptive pills
Emotional disturbances
Anorexia nervosa
Infection
Cysts or tumours of the ovary
Endocrine diseases
Drugs

Pregnancy

Amenorrhoea occurs during pregnancy and persists during lactation.

Menopause

The menopause occurs at 45–55 years. Menstruation may (a) end suddenly, (b) get less and less at each period until it stops, or (c) occur at longer and longer intervals until it stops.

Contraceptive pills

Contraceptive pills contain synthetic oestrogen and progestogen and act on the ovaries or hypothalamus.

Emotional disturbances

A temporary cessation of menstruation, especially within two or three years of onset, can be caused by emotional disturbances and changes of environment. Amenorrhoea can occur during any psychosis.

Anorexia nervosa

This is a disease of young women in which they starve themselves, become emaciated, and develop amenorrhoea, anaemia and excessive hairiness.

Infection

Amenorrhoea can be due to any chronic infection, especially tuberculosis. The patient is likely to complain of tiredness and malaise, to have a raised temperature, and to have a ESR (Erythrocyte Sedimentation Rate) above the normal of 0–7 mm in 1 hour.

Cysts or tumours of the ovary

Amenorrhoea can be due to a cyst or tumour of the ovary, especially:

polycystic ovaries (Stein-Leventhal syndrome),
follicle cyst,
corpus luteum cyst,
granulosa cell tumour,
theca cell tumour,
arrhenoblastoma.

Endocrine diseases

Amenorrhoea can occur in:

gigantism,
acromegaly,
Simmonds' disease,
hyperthyroidism (thyrotoxicosis),
hypothyroidism (cretinism, myxoedema),
diabetes mellitus,
Addison's disease.

Drugs

Amenorrhoea can be caused by drugs which interfere with hypothalamic function and so prevent the formation of sex hormones. The drugs are:

phenothiazines
reserpine and ganglion-blocking agents.

MENORRHAGIA

Menorrhagia is excessive menstrual loss. Women vary in the

amount they lose, and menorrhagia is present when a woman loses more than she considers normal for herself.

Causes of menorrhagia

Endometriosis
Fibroid tumour
Endometrial polyp
Chronic inflammatory pelvic disease
Disease of the blood
Thyroid dysfunction
Unknown

Endometriosis

In this condition menorrhagia is associated with dysmenorrhoea and dyspareunia (pain on sexual intercourse). The endometrium (inner layer of the uterus) is thickened, raised into polypoid masses, and likely to contain cysts. On vaginal examination the uterus is found to be enlarged and tender.

Fibroid tumour

A fibroid tumour is a benign tumour of the uterus and composed of muscle and fibrous tissue. In addition to the heavy loss, the period of menstruation is likely to be prolonged. Menorrhagia is due to a fibroid enlarging the cavity of the uterus, exposing a larger bleeding area, and producing increased vascularity of the uterus.

Endometrial polyp

Menorrhagia, bleeding between periods and a discharge can be due to an endometrial polyp. This is an outgrowth of endometrium which projects into the uterine cavity, and if it has a long stalk it can appear at the opening of the cervix into the vagina.

Chronic inflammatory pelvic disease

Menorrhagia can be due to any chronic inflammatory disease of the pelvic organs:

> chronic gonococcal salpingitis,
> puerperal salpingitis,
> pelvic tuberculosis.

(a) *Chronic gonococcal salpingitis* follows an acute gonococcal salpingitis, which is characterized by lower abdominal pain, fever and a discharge. Untreated or inadequately treated, a chronic inflammation occurs which produces menorrhagia, dysmenorrhoea, dyspareunia (pain on sexual intercourse), lower abdominal pain, general ill-health and often infertility.

(b) *Puerperal salpingitis* is similar to gonococcal salpingitis, but is due to invasion of the ovarian tubes and pelvis by *streptococci* during the puerperium (the period after childbirth).

(c) *Pelvic tuberculosis* is secondary to tuberculosis elsewhere in the body. A chronic low-grade infection with abscesses and adhesions is produced.

Diseases of the blood

Menorrhagia can occur in any of the blood diseases of which bleeding is a feature:

> purpura,
> scurvy.

Thyroid dysfunction

Menorrhagia can occur in myxoedema and hyperthyroidism (thyrotoxicosis).

Unknown

For some cases of menorrhagia no cause can be found.

IRREGULAR BLEEDING

Irregular bleeding can occur between periods or after the menopause.

Causes of irregular bleeding

Carcinoma of cervix of uterus
Cervical erosion
Chronic cervicitis
Cervical polyp
Ulceration of vagina
Carcinoma of body of uterus
Drugs

Carcinoma of cervix of uterus

Bleeding from a carcinoma of the cervix of the uterus occurs between periods or after the menopause. The patient is usually 40–50 years old and usually has had children. The carcinoma appears as a soft, ulcerated, bleeding mass in the cervix, which it gradually destroys; when infection of it has occurred there is an offensive, blood-stained discharge.

Cervical erosion and chronic cervicitis

These non-malignant diseases of the cervix cause irregular bleeding and a discharge. An erosion is a bright red degenerated area, secondary to a cervical discharge. In cervicitis the mucous membrane is thickened and polyps and cysts may be present.

Cervical polyp

There is a small soft pink projection from the inner surface of the cervix, and is usually secondary to cervicitis. It can project through the external os of the cervix. It causes bleeding and a discharge.

Ulceration of vagina

Bleeding can be due to ulceration of the vagina by a foreign body, of which the most common is a pessary. Ulceration can be due to an attempt to procure abortion.

Carcinoma of body of uterus

A blood-stained discharge is the first symptom of carcinoma of the body of the uterus; when infection of the tumour occurs it has an offensive smell. Any bleeding is not usually profuse. Slight abdominal pain may occur, and more severe pain when the tumour has spread beyond the uterus. The patient is usually 50–60 years old.

Drugs

Irregular bleeding from the endometrium can occur as a side effect of hormones used for gynaecological conditions:

> oestrogens,
> progestogens.

Headache, vomiting, a 'blown up' feeling of the abdomen, and depression are other side effects.

37. Vaginal Discharge

The normal white discharge is due to secretion from glands in the cervix of the uterus; it contains cells shed from the vaginal epithelium.

Leucorrhoea is excessive but otherwise normal discharge which occurs in some women.

Causes of vaginal discharge

Trichomonas infection
Candida albicans infection
Gonorrhoea
Foreign body in vagina
Senile vaginitis
Chronic cervicitis and cervical erosion
Carcinoma of vagina
Carcinoma of cervix or body of uterus
Senile endometritis
Faecal fistula
Pelvic abscess

Trichomonas infection

A thin, yellowish-green, offensive discharge containing tiny bubbles is produced by infection of the vagina by *Trichomonas vaginalis*, a microscopic pear-shaped organism transmitted by sexual intercourse. It can cause irritation of the vulva and upper thighs.

Candida albicans infection

A white curdy discharge which partly adheres to the wall of the vagina and intense irritation is caused by infection by *Candida albicans*, a yeast. It is liable to occur especially during pregnancy and in diabetic patients with glycosuria.

Gonorrhoea

A mucopurulent discharge is produced by gonococcal infection of the cervix of the uterus and of the urethra. In some women the discharge is slight and not enough to warn the woman that she has been infected. Vulval irritation and painful micturition can occur.

Foreign body in vagina

A purulent discharge can be produced by a foreign body, such as a Tampax or a pessary, in the vagina. The discharge can become offensive if the foreign body has been there a long time.

Senile vaginitis

A blood-stained purulent discharge with vulval irritation and painful micturition occurs with senile vaginitis, an atrophic and inflammatory condition of the vagina liable to occur in old women.

Chronic cervicitis and cervical erosion

A profuse mucopurulent discharge is produced by chronic cervicitis and a cervical erosion. It is likely to be associated with frequency of micturition, pain in the back and lower abdominal discomfort.

Carcinoma of the vagina

A blood-stained discharge is likely in carcinoma of the vagina, a rare tumour which occurs usually in old age.

Carcinoma of cervix or body of uterus

A blood-stained discharge, in addition to haemorrhage, occurs in both these conditions, and in later stages of the disease it becomes offensive.

Senile endometritis

A blood-stained discharge follows ulceration of the endometrium in this condition, an atrophy and inflammation of the endometrium liable to occur in old age.

Faecal fistula

Pus and faeces can be passed into the vagina through a faecal fistula, when diseased bowel and vagina become adherent to one another. This can occur in diverticulitis, carcinoma of the large intestine, carcinoma of the uterus, etc.

Pelvic abscess

Pus can be discharged into the vagina from a pelvic abscess. The pelvic abscess can be due to appendicitis, salpingitis, puerperal sepsis, etc.

38. Pain and Lumps in the Breast

Pain in the breast is called mastalgia. Any woman who has pain or a lump in the breast is likely to think she has cancer. There are many other causes.

Causes of pain and lumps in the breast

Pregnancy
Trauma
Pubertal mastitis
Breast abscess
Cyst
Fibroadenoma
Fibrosis of breast
Carcinoma of breast
Mammary duct ectasia
Sclerosing adenosis
Cyclical pronounced mastalgia
Tietze syndrome

Pregnancy

Enlargement of the breasts in pregnancy can cause pain.

Trauma

Pain in the breast can be produced by a blow severe enough to produce a haematoma or fat necrosis. A haematoma may be felt as a lump. Pain is sometimes experienced in a surgical scar, sometimes years after operation.

Pubertal mastitis

A non-suppurative mastitis at puberty can cause pain and swelling. It is usually unilateral, can be bilateral, and resolves spontaneously in 2–6 weeks.

Breast abscess

A breast abscess can follow infection of the breast by a pyogenic micro-organisms. It is most common in lactating women, but it can occur in some who are not, possibly as a result of infection of a haematoma. The usual signs of an acute abscess are present.

Cyst

A cyst of the breast appears as a painless, smooth, rounded, well limited lump. It is soft when it is not distended with fluid, hard when it is or when it is a long-standing cyst with thick fibrous walls. There may be a single cyst or a group of several. Occasionally signs of inflammation are present.

Fibroadenoma of breast

This appears in adolescence or early adult life as a painless, smooth, freely movable lump, which slips away from the fingers when it is being palpated.

Fibrosis of breast

This presents as a painless lump, which being somewhat fixed in the breast tissue and not having a clearly limited edge may be mistaken for a carcinoma.

Carcinoma of breast

Pain can be the first sign of a cancer of the breast and is usually localized to the site of the growth. There may be a definite hard tumour or a diffuse lumpiness of the breast. The lump can be attached to the skin or to the pectoral sheath. The nipple may be retracted and there may be a blood-stained discharge with it. If the cancer has spread to the axillary glands, it may be palpable as hard rounded lumps.

Mammary duct ectasia

This is a dilatation of the terminal mammary ducts beneath

the nipple and areola. It occurs in the second half of life. It produces a lump and pain. The lump may be mistaken clinically for a carcinoma, especially as the nipple can be retracted or a discharge from it occur. Pain can often be precisely located and in some women is worse in winter.

Sclerosing adenosis

This is a condition in which there is an enlargement of the acini of the glands and a secondary fibrosis. It usually occurs in middle age. There is persistent pain and lumpiness or a lump in the breast. The lump is not attached to the skin or to deeper tissues. There may be a discharge from the nipple.

Cyclical pronounced mastalgia

In this condition a pain in the breast occurs or is exacerbated during the premenstrual period and is absent or slight during the rest of the menstrual cycle. The pain can occur simultaneously in both breasts and be felt throughout the breast. The patients sometimes describe the pain as feeling as if the breasts were distended with milk. The cause is thought to be hormonal.

Tietze syndrome

This is a condition in which an aching pain in the breast is sometimes associated with a tender and enlarged junction of a rib with its costal cartilage. Some women locate the pain in the chest, not in the breast.

39. Itching

Itching (pruritus) is the senation transmitted from 'itch points' in the skin along sensory nerve fibres to the thalamus and the sensory areas of the cerebral cortex. The 'itch points' are concentrations of sensitive nerve endings. Itching can be temperarily relieved by scratching or rubbing, possibly because the transmission of other sensory stimuli blocks out the impulses of itching. Itching is usually worse when a person is not concentrating at work or play; it is often worse when he is in bed and can interfere with sleep. Some skin diseases produce itching in some people and not in others.

Itching can occur generally all over the skin or locally, i.e. in one part of the skin only.

Causes of itching

Parasites and insects
Allergies and irritants
Fungus infections
Heat and cold
Other skin diseases
General conditions and diseases of the body

Parasites

Itching can be due to:

scabies,
lice,
fleas and other biting insects.

(a) *Scabies* is such a common cause of intense itching that it is commonly known as 'the itch'. It is one of the first conditions to be considered when a patient complains of itching.

Scabies is due to the invasion of the skin by the female of a small mite, which lay its eggs in its burrows. The burrows are visible as thin grey lines. The usual sites of infection are the clefts between the fingers, the front of the wrist, the inner side of the elbow, under the breasts, and on the external genitalia.

(b) *Lice.* Infection by lice, which most commonly occurs in the scalp and the pubic hair, causes itching. The lice and their eggs (nits) can be found in the hair. People who have been infected for years may not feel any discomfort.

(c) *Fleas and other biting insects.* Fleas and other biting insects cause itching at the site of the bites.

Allergies and irritants

(a) *Eczema* is an allergic reaction of the skin to an internal or external stimulus and commonly causes itching. The condition is recognized by the typical rash on the face, forearms, legs and flexure areas. The skin becomes reddened and papules and vesicles appear. Lichenification, a thickness and roughness of the skin, appears in chronic cases as a result of scratching and rubbing.

(b) *Urticaria* is an allergic reaction of the skin due to internal or external causes. Papules and weals appear. The papules itch intensely.

(c) *Irritants*, such as powders or liquids, can cause itching in people whose skin is sensitive to them. Exposure to radiation can cause itching.

Fungus infection

Itching is caused by fungus infections of the skin. Common sites of infection are between the fourth and fifth toes, in the groin, under the breasts, in the anal and vulval regions. Between the toes the skin becomes thickened and sodden. On other sites, vesicles appear on an inflamed base. The itching can be intense.

Heat and cold

(a) *Sunburn.* Itching occurs in recently sunburned skin.

(b) *Prickly heat.* This is a hot itching condition of the skin liable to occur in newcomers to the tropics or in people exposed to sunlight for long periods.

(c) *Chilblains.* Chilblains itch or burn intensely. They are a result of arteriolar spasm and venous stagnation in the toes, fingers and nose.

Other skin diseases

Itching can occur in:

seborrhoea,　　　　　　　psoriasis,
lichen planus,　　　　　　pityriasis rosea,
dermatitis herpetiformis,　herpes zoster,
herpes simplex,　　　　　chickenpox,
vaccinia.

(a) *Seborrhoea.* In the early stages of seborrhoeic dermatitis, in which there is an excessive secretion of sebum in the hairy parts of the skin, dandruff appears in the scalp and other affected parts and causes local itching.

(b) *Psoriasis.* Psoriasis, a recurrent disease of the skin of unknown cause, is characterized by raised reddish patches with sharp edges and silvery scaling on the surface of the patches. Several forms of the disease occur. It is peculiar in that it causes itching in some patients and none in others.

(c) *Lichen planus.* Lichen planus is a disease of unknown causes in which flat violet papules appear on the skin and white papules on the mucous membrane of the mouth, fauces, vagina and rectum. Severe itching occurs in some patients but not in others.

(d) *Pityriasis rosea.* Pityriasis rosea is thought to be a response to a viral infection of the upper respiratory tract. A pink 'herald patch' appears and is followed by a crop of pink spots and papules which last for a few weeks. Generalized itching occurs all the time or only after a hot bath.

(e) *Dermatitis herpetiformis.* In this disease of unknown origin, papules, vesicles and bullae develop in any part of the skin and most commonly on the buttocks, genitalia, elbows and back. Affected areas itch intensely.

(f) *Herpes simplex*. Herpes simplex, a recurrent viral infection, produces crops of vesicles and around the mouth, inside the mouth, on the fingers and elsewhere. Itching sometimes occurs before the vesicles appear.

(g) *Herpes zoster*. Herpes zoster is an erythematous and vesicular rash occuring in the area of skin supplied by a sensory nerve, usually on the face or trunk. Itching and pain in the affected areas are common before, during and sometime for years after the appearance of the lesions in the skin. It occurs in middle-aged or old people as the result of a reactivation of the virus of chickenpox, which has laid latent in the tissues since an attack in childhood.

(h) *Vaccinia*. Itching can occur at the site of the vaccination against smallpox.

(i) *Chickenpox*. Itching of the skin is a common feature of chickenpox.

General conditions and diseases of the body

Itching can be a feature of some conditions and diseases without any apparent disease of the skin.
   These conditions include:

> pregnancy,
> diseases of the liver,
> diseases of the blood,
> carcinoma of internal organs,
> metabolic and endocrine diseases,
> malabsorption
> worm infection,
> old age,
> diseases of the kidney,
> Hodgkin's disease,
> diseases of connective tissue.

(a) *Pregnancy*. Itching is common in pregnancy. It may be general or limited to the skin of the abdomen. In the later stages of pregnancy some women develop *prurigo*, which is characterized by itchy papules on the upper arms, trunk and legs. Itching in the vulval region would suggest a local infection by *Candida* (a mould) or a trichomonal infection of the vagina.

(b) *Old age.* Itching is common in old age. Usually no cause can be found. It may be general or limited to a small area of skin between the scapulae.

(c) *Diseases of the liver.* Itching is common in some diseases of the liver and is usually worst on the forearms, chest and legs. It is due to a rise in the level of bile acids in the blood as a result of obstruction to the flow of bile, either within the small ducts in the liver or in the bile ducts outside it, and is relieved by the oral administration of cholestyramine, which lowers the bile acid level in the blood. Itching is not a feature of severe jaundice, in which the production of bile acids is reduced.

(d) *Diseases of the kidney.* Itching is common in chronic renal disease. In renal failure the skin as well as itching is liable to become dry.

(e) *Disease of the blood.* Severe itching and burning are features of lymphatic leukaemia and polycythaemia vera. In *lymphatic leukaemia* the lymph nodes are enlarged and there is a great increase in the number of lymphacytes in the blood. In *polycythaemia vera* the patient is a deep red colour, has an enlarged spleen and sometimes an enlarged liver; his blood shows a great increase in the number of red cells.

(f) *Hodgkin's disease* (lymphadenoma). Severe itching and burning can be a feature of Hodgkin's disease. Itching can be the first feature and is sometimes limited to the legs. Other features are enlarged lymph nodes and an enlarged spleen and liver.

(g) *Carcinoma of internal organs.* Slight itching is common and urticarial weals can develop in cases of carcinoma of any internal organ.

(h) *Metabolic and endocrine diseases.* In *diabetes mellitus* generalized itching or pruritus ani and vulvae can occur. Itching can occur in *hypothyroidism*, less commonly in *hyperthyroidism*, and sometimes in *gout.*

(i) *Malabsorption.* Itching is a feature of malabsorption syndromes, in which owing to disease or surgical removal of the small intestine, there is an inadequate absorption of foodstuffs, minerals and vitamins.

(j) *Diseases of connective tissue.* Itching can occur in *dermatomyositis*, a collagen disease characterized by rashes, muscular pain and myocarditis, and sometimes in *systemic lupus erythematosus*, a chronic collagen disease with degenerative changes in many tissues and organs.

(k) *Worm infection.* Itching can occur in *hookworm infection*, especially in the feet through the skin of which the larvae of the worm invade the body, and in *onochocerciasis*, an infection by a filarial worm.

PRURITUS ANI

Itching in the anal region usually occurs without any physical signs, except those of the basic cause and those produced by scratching. It is more common in men than women.

Causes of pruritus ani

Lack of cleanliness
Threadworms
Haemorrhoids
Anal fissure
Pubic lice
Fungus infection
Drugs (phenolphthalein; wide-spectrum antibiotics, which encourage fungus growth; locally applied drugs)
Vitamin A deficiency
Emotional causes

PRURITUS VULVAE

Itching of the vulva usually occurs without any physical signs, except those of the basic cause and those produced by scratching.

Causes of pruritus vulvae

Lack of cleanliness
Vaginal discharge from any cause
Pregnancy
Glycosuria in diabetes mellitus
Threadworms
Pubic lice
Sensitivity to vaginal douches and local applications
Drugs (oral contraceptives; wide-spectrum antibiotics, which encourage fungus growth)
Emotional causes

Index